Pocket Guide to
Electrocardiography

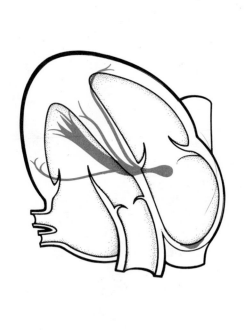

Pocket Guide to Electrocardiography

Mary Boudreau Conover, R.N., B.S.

Instructor of Intermediate and Advanced Arrhythmia
Workshops, West Hills Hospital, Canoga Park, California;
Education Consultant, Center for Diagnosis and Treatment
of Cardiac Arrhythmias, Holy Cross Hospital,
Mission Hills, California

REVISED EDITION

with 367 illustrations

The C. V. Mosby Company

St. Louis • Baltimore • Toronto   1986

MOSBY

A TRADITION OF PUBLISHING EXCELLENCE

Cover photograph © G. Robert Bishop, 1985

REVISED EDITION

Printed in the United States of America

The C.V. Mosby Company
11830 Westline Industrial Drive, St. Louis, Missouri 63146

Library of Congress Cataloging in Publication Data

Conover, Mary Boudreau.
  Pocket guide to electrocardiography.

  Includes index.
  1. Electrocardiography—Handbooks, manuals, etc.
2. Heart—Diseases—Diagnosis—Handbooks, manuals, etc.
3. Arrhythmia—Diagnosis—Handbooks, manuals, etc.
4. Cardiovascular disease nursing—Handbooks, manuals,
etc. I. Title. [DNLM: 1. Electrocardiography—
handbooks. 2. Electrocardiography—nurses' instruction.
WG 39 C753p]
RC683.5.E5C646 1986   616.1'207547   85-18753
ISBN 0-8016-1049-4

C/D/D 9 8 7 6 5 4   04/B/548

Dedication

To those from whom I have learned—through their writings
or through their personal instruction and advice:

Henry J.L. Marriott, M.D.
Hein J.J. Wellens, M.D.
Sarko M. Tilkian, M.D.
Ara G. Tilkian, M.D.
David C. Gadsby, M.A., Ph.D.
Paul F. Cranefield, M.D., Ph.D.
Albert L. Waldo, M.D.
William P. Nelson, M.D.
Demetrius Sodi-Pallaris, M.D.
Brian F. Hoffman, M.D.
Robert H. Anderson, M.D.
Maricio B. Rosenbaum, M.D.
John J. Gallagher, M.D.

Editor Nancy L. Mullins
Developmental Editor Thomas A. Lochhaas
Assistant Editors Maureen Slaten, Bess Arends
Manuscript Editors Carol Sullivan Wiseman, Stephen C. Hetager
Designer Diane M. Beasley
Production Jeanne A. Gulledge

Mosby Reviewers

Foreword

In 1962, Dr. Hughes Day opened the first cardiac care unit—
at Bethany Hospital in Kansas City. The intervening years
have seen a remarkable growth in the number of these special-
care units, and most community hospitals boast such facilities
today. In most units, the real "coronary care–taker" is the
nurse and not the physician. Thus, it has become increasingly
important for the CCU nurse to be familiar with the array of
electrocardiographic abnormalities that may be encountered in
cardiac patients.

Mary Conover provides a thorough, clear, and concise review of such abnormalities in this "pocket book." It is richly
illustrated and replete with practical suggestions, and it con-
stitutes a stimulating review of current concepts of diagnosis
and therapy.

William P. Nelson, M.D.
Professor of Medicine,
University of South Florida College of Medicine,
Tampa, Florida;
Director, Cardiac Care Unit,
James A. Haley Veterans Hospital,
Tampa, Florida

Preface

This book provides key information for the rapid recognition of arrhythmias and abnormal 12-lead electrocardiograms. The format is uniform and concise for rapid reference; the information is up to date. Each abnormal tracing or 12-lead ECG is described, and its pathophysiology and mechanism are explained; ECG characteristics, causes, and types of treatment are listed and distinguishing features emphasized. Nursing implications and differential diagnoses are developed, and a helpful and complete list of variations is provided.

Invasive cardiology has revitalized the surface ECG and established it as an accurate tool in the differential diagnosis of arrhythmogenic mechanisms and the location of myocardial infarction. It has confirmed and firmly established the traditional ECG clues and has given us new ones. Thus the surface ECG is more important than ever before, and we are reminded that its usefulness and accuracy are stifled by slavish devotion to one lead and by overdependence on invasive diagnostic tools or computer diagnosis.

I am grateful to Dr. William P. Nelson for his critical review of the manuscript.

Mary Boudreau Conover

Contents

Principles of Electrocardiography

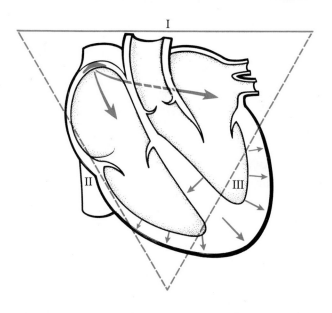

The Electrocardiogram

The electrocardiograph is the instrument that records the electrical activity of the heart, and the electrocardiogram (ECG) is the record of the activity. Electrodes of opposite polarity are placed on the skin at opposite poles of the electrical field; these two electrodes constitute a bipolar lead. One positive electrode and a reference point constitute a unipolar lead. The leads are attached to an amplifier within an oscilloscope or strip recorder. The interpretation of this record is the basis for the ECG diagnosis of arrhythmias.

The 12 Leads

There are six limb leads, three bipolar and three unipolar, and six precordial leads in the standard 12-lead ECG. The precordial leads are unipolar. The limb leads provide information about superior, inferior, right, and left forces; the precordial leads provide information about anterior, posterior, right, and left forces.

The Three Bipolar Limb Leads

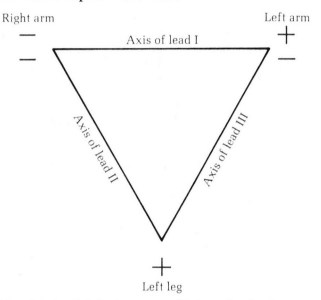

Three bipolar limb leads compose Einthoven's triangle.

The axis of lead I is from shoulder to shoulder. The negative electrode is on the right arm, and the positive on the left.

The axis of lead II is from the right shoulder to the left leg. The negative electrode is on the right arm and the positive on the left.

The axis of lead III is from the left shoulder to the left leg. The negative electrode is on the left arm, and the positive on the left leg.

These electrodes are all about equally distant from the heart; thus the triangle they form is truly *equilateral*.

The Three Unipolar Limb Leads

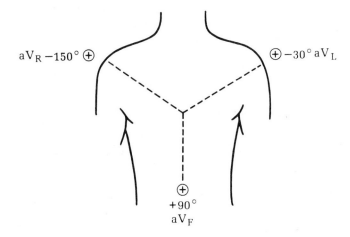

$aV_R -150° \oplus$ $\oplus -30° \, aV_L$

$\oplus$
$+90°$
aV_F

If the two arm electrodes and the left leg electrode are connected to a central terminal through resistances of 5000 ohms each, the sum of the potentials is considered to be zero. The positive exploring electrodes can be paired with this indifferent reference point to permit the use of unipolar leads (aV_R, aV_L, or aV_F).

The Precordial Leads

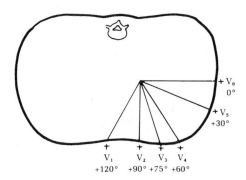

$+ V_6$
$0°$

$+ V_5$
$+30°$

$+$ $+$ $+$ $+$
V_1 V_2 V_3 V_4
$+120°$ $+90°$ $+75°$ $+60°$

The six principal precordial leads, V_1 to V_6, are unipolar leads whose axes are from the positive electrodes on the chest wall to a zero potential reference point in the center of the electrical field. The electrode positions curve around the thorax over the heart from the right ventricle across the septum to the lateral wall of the left ventricle. Placement of the precordial electrodes is as follows:

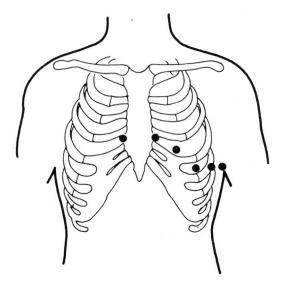

V_1 and V_2: On either side of the sternum at the fourth interspace

V_4: Midclavicular line, fifth interspace

V_3: Midway between V_4 and V_2

V_5 and V_6: On the same level with V_4 in the anterior and midaxillary lines, respectively

Placement of additional helpful precordial leads is as follows:

MCL_1 (bipolar lead that simulates V_1): Positive electrode in same position as V_1; negative electrode, left midclavicle

V_{3R} to V_{6R}: Right precordial leads (unipolar) that correspond to left precordial leads

Instant-to-instant Cardiac Vectors and Electrical Axis

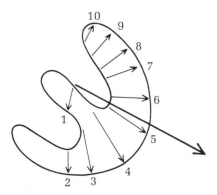

The arrows in the figure above represent the instant-to-instant cardiac vectors, which are numbered in the order of their completion. The sum of all of the cardiac vectors generated during the cardiac cycle is called the electrical axis and is represented by the largest arrow. Even though the currents begin almost simultaneously at the endocardium in both ventricles, the currents in the thicker left-ventricular wall take longer and are stronger than those in the right-ventricular wall. Thus left-ventricular forces dominate those of the right ventricle.

In the critical care setting, determinations of electrical axis are made to assess the fascicles of the left bundle branch and to differentiate between ventricular aberrancy and ventricular ectopy. This determination can be made by any one of several methods with leads I, II, and aV_F being the keys to instant recognition; for example, I and II will tell you when the axis is the extreme left (> -30 degrees) and I and aV_F when it is to the left (>0 degrees).

Main Current Flow and the Axis of a Lead

The lead axis is an imaginary line drawn between the two electrodes or between an electrode and a reference point.

When the main current flow is parallel with the axis of a lead, the resulting complex is either the most positive or the most negative deflection of all.

When the main current flow is perpendicular to the axis of a lead, an equiphasic deflection is drawn. In Fig. 1-1 note that it does not matter in which direction this current is going; as long as it is perpendicular to the axis of the lead, an equiphasic deflection results.

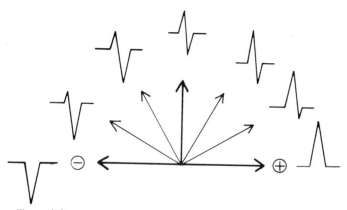

Figure 1-1

A number of mean vectors are combined here to illustrate the possible different complexes. A mean vector that is perpendicular to the lead axis produces an equiphasic deflection. A mean vector on the positive side of the perpendicular and yet not parallel with the lead axis produces a complex that is mostly positive. However, if the mean vector is on the negative side of the perpendicular and yet not parallel with the lead axis, the complex is mostly negative.

An Easy Two-step Method of Axis Determination

Fig. 1-2 is an example of the easy two-step method of axis determination. In the first step, look for an equiphasic deflection; it shows that current flow is perpendicular to that lead axis. In this case it is found in aV_R. However, this is incomplete information because the main current flow may be in either direction. So, in the second step, look at the lead whose axis is parallel to this current flow; it shows the direction the current is flowing. In this case that lead is III. Since the complex in III is negative, current is flowing toward the negative electrode of lead III (left axis deviation of -60 degrees). This simple exercise shows that this is a left axis, although you may not yet be able to pinpoint the degree of the axis. However, in time you can become adept at determing this degree.

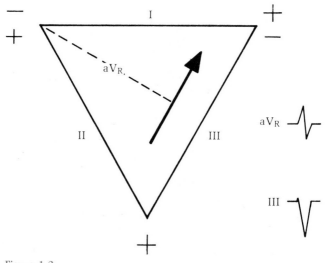

Figure 1-2
Deflections in aV_R and III when the axis is -60 degrees (LAD).

Recognizing Axis at a Glance

Normal		Left		Extreme left		Right	
−30 to +110°		>0°		>−30°		>+110°	
I	II	I	AVF	I	II	I	II

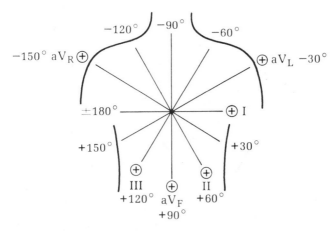

The Hexaxial Figure

When a more precise determination of axis is needed, the hexaxial figure is used. In the figure above all of the frontal plane lead axes are drawn through a central point. Note that each lead axis is a 30-degree increment so that with lead I at 0 degrees, aV_R, II, and aV_F are on the plus side at 30, 60, and 90 degrees; on the negative side are aV_L, III, and the negative pole of aV_F at 30, 60, and 90 degrees.

The Normal ECG in the 12 Leads

Understanding the 12-lead ECG involves many concepts, beginning with the limb and precordial leads and electrical axis, and then the components of the normal ECG as they should look in the 12 leads. Since much more is involved in a complete understanding of the 12-lead ECG, all of the following will be addressed in this book:

AV conduction
Intraventricular conduction
Initial forces
Anterior and posterior forces
Bundle-branch block
Hemiblock
Aberrancy
Wolff-Parkinson-White (WPW) syndrome
Lown-Ganong-Levine (LGL) syndrome
Myocardial infarction
Chamber enlargement

ECG Grid Paper

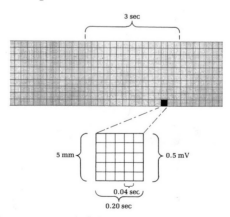

Time is measured on the horizontal plane. Each small square is 1 mm in length and represents 0.04 sec. Each larger square is 5 mm long and represents 0.2 sec.

Voltage is measured on the vertical plane, and 1 mV is equal to 10 mm in the standardized ECG.

ECG Components (Fig. 1-3)

P Wave

- Mechanism: Reflects atrial depolarization
- Duration: Not over 0.11 sec
- Amplitude: Not more than 3 mm
- Shape: No notching or peaking
- Polarity:
  Positive in I, II, aV_F, V_4 to V_6
  Negative in aV_R
  Positive, negative, or diphasic in III, aV_L, and V_1 to V_3
  If diphasic, the negative component is last and not excessively broad or deep.
- Clinical significance of abnormalities:
  Inversion where it should be upright—premature atrial complexes (PACs) or premature junctional complexes (PJCs)

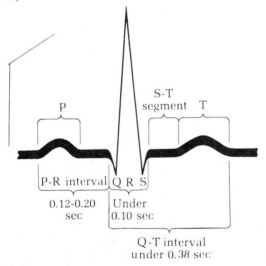

Figure 1-3
Diagrammatic representation of the ECG and its intervals.

Increased amplitude—atrial hypertrophy or dilation, usually secondary to atrioventicular (AV) valve disease, hypertension, cor pulmonale, or congenital heart disease

Increased width and notching—left-atrial enlargement or diseased atria

Diphasic with the negative component excessively wide in II or V_1—left atrial enlargement

Peaking that is taller in I than III—right atrial overload

Absent P waves—SA block or a junctional rhythm

QRS Complex

- Mechanism: Reflects ventricular depolarization
- Duration: Not over 0.10 sec
- Amplitude (total): wide normal limits
  Not less than 5 mm in II, III, aV_F, V_1, and V_6
  Not less than 7 mm in V_2 and V_5
  Not less than 9 mm in V_3 and V_4
  Not over 25 to 30 mm in the precordial leads
- Shape: R waves are positive; Q and S waves are negative.
  A Q wave comes before the R; an S wave follows the R.
  QRS is a generic term; the exact shape is described by using upper and lower case letters, which indicate the relative sizes of the components (Fig. 1-4).
- Polarity:
  Initial forces (septal)
    Narrow q of 1 to 2 mm in V_6, I, and aV_L
    Narrow r in V_1 may normally be absent
  Terminal forces (left ventricular)
    S in V_1
    R in V_6

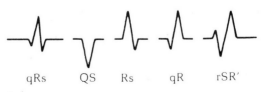

qRs   QS   Rs   qR   rSR′

Figure 1-4
QRS deflections.

- Clinical significance of abnormalities:

  Excessive width reflects intraventricular conduction problems.

  Excessive height may indicate hypertrophy or enlargement of the ventricle.

  Low voltage may indicate diffuse coronary disease, cardiac failure, pericardial effusion, myxedema, primary amyloidosis, emphysema, obesity, or generalized edema.

  The presence or absence of Q waves is judged in the clinical setting.

T Wave

- Mechanism: Reflects ventricular repolarization
- Amplitude: Not more than 5 mm in standard leads and 10 mm in precordial leads
- Shape: Rounded and asymmetrical (notching normal in children)
- Polarity: Positive in I, II, V_3 to V_6

  Negative in aV_R

  Positive in aV_L and aV_F but may be negative if QRS is < 5 mm

  Varies in III, V_1, and V_2
- Clinical significance of abnormalities:

  Inversion may indicate diffuse myocardial ischemia or subendocardial infarction, but is not specific.

  Notching, other than in children, may indicate pericarditis.

  Sharp and pointed shape may indicate myocardial infarction.

  Increased amplitude suggests myocardial infarction or hyperkalemia; also myocardial ischemia and ventricular overload.

ST Segment

- Mechanism: Represents early stage of ventricular repolarization
- Polarity:

  May be elevated slightly (1 mm) in I, II, and III, and 2 mm in the precordial leads

  Normally not depressed more than 0.5 mm anywhere

  May be depressed as much as 4 mm in precordial leads in young black men (early repolarization syndrome)

- Clinical significance of abnormalities:
  Significant displacement—coronary artery disease (marked elevation suggests myocardial infarction, marked depression at rest suggests ischemia or subendocardial infarction and depression during stress tests suggests occult coronary artery disease).
  Digitalis causes typical depression.
  Temporary elevation may result from direct current (DC) cardioversion.

PR Interval

- Mechanism: Represents AV conduction time
- Duration: 0.12 to 0.20 sec
- Clinical significance of abnormalities:
  Too short with a normal QRS—Lown-Ganong-Levine syndrome
  Too short with a broad QRS—Wolff-Parkinson-White syndrome
  Too long—AV block or beta blockers

QT Interval

- Mechanism: Represents repolarization time
- Duration: Less than half the preceeding RR interval as a general rule
- Clinical significance of abnormalities:
  QT lengthening may be idiopathic or caused by drugs (quinidine, procainamide, disopyramide, or amiodarone), electrolyte imbalance (hypokalemia), cerebrovascular disease, hypothermia, or bradycardia.

U Wave

- Mechanism: Unknown
- Amplitude: Low voltage
- Polarity: Same as T wave
- Clinical significance of abnormalities:
  Hypokalemia (tall U wave)
  Reversed polarity in ischemia, left ventricular overload as a result of hypertension, aortic or mitral regurgitation, and left coronary artery disease (at rest)

Calculation of Heart Rate

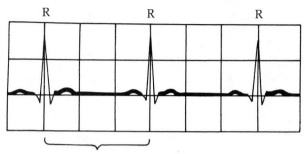

$300 \div 3 = 100/\text{min} = \text{Heart rate}$

When the rhythm is regular, heart rate can be determined at a glance by counting the large squares between R waves and dividing into 300.

When the rhythm is irregular, count the R waves in a 6-sec strip and multiply by 10.

Arrhythmias Originating in the Sinus Node

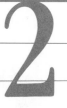

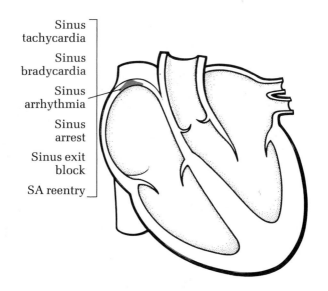

Sinus tachycardia

Sinus bradycardia

Sinus arrhythmia

Sinus arrest

Sinus exit block

SA reentry

The arrhythmias originating in the sinus (or sinoatrial [SA]) node are sinus tachycardia, sinus bradycardia, sinus arrhythmia, SA block, SA nodal reentry, sick sinus syndrome, and sinus arrest. In all of these arrhythmias, the sinus node is the pacemaker of the heart. However, its rate is too fast, too slow, irregular, or inconsistent.

Anatomy and Physiology

The SA node is located in the wall of the right atrium, adjacent to the superior vena cava. Fig. 2-1 shows that the body

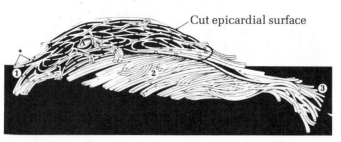

Figure 2-1
A wax model of the human sinus node.
(From Truex, R.C. In Wellens, H.J.J., Lie, K.I., and Janse, M.J., editors:
The conduction system of the heart, Hingham, Mass., 1976, Martinus Nijhoff
Publishers.)

of the SA node blends with perinodal fibers, which in turn blend with atrial tissue. The SA node has only slow calcium-sodium channel action potentials; therefore conduction velocity through the node is normally slow.

Sinus Tachycardia

Sinus tachycardia is a regular sinus rhythm of more than 100 beats/min. It may be one of the first signs of congestive heart failure, cardiogenic shock, pulmonary embolism, or infarct extension.

Pathophysiology and Mechanism

There is usually no pathology in sinus tachycardia unless it occurs as part of the sick sinus syndrome. It is either the normal response to the demand for increased blood flow, in which case the vagal stimulation is less and sympathetic stimulation more, resulting in enhanced automaticity in the node, or it is caused by drugs.

ECG Characteristics

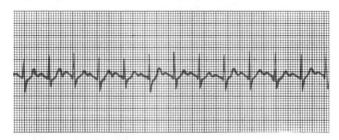

Rate: >100 beats/min

Rhythm: Regular

PR interval: Normal, although the PR may be too long or too short because of other conditions. All of the P waves are the same shape and are upright in leads I, II, aV$_F$, and V$_4$ to V$_6$.

QRS complex: Normal, although the QRS may be prolonged as a result of other conditions

Distinguishing features: Rate, rhythm, and uniform shape of the P waves

Causes

- Drugs, such as atropine, isoproterenol (Isuprel), quinidine, and epinephrine (Adrenalin)
- Exercise, emotions, fever, or pain
- Hyperthyroidism
- Conditions involving increased sympathetic stimulation

Nursing Implications

In the presence of acute ischemic changes, an increase in heart rate, even from a physiological sinus mechanism or the administration of atropine, may trigger ventricular arrhythmias because of an enhancement of the ischemia, a lowering of the fibrillation threshold, and a greater dispersion of refractoriness.

The rapid rate is quickly diagnosed if the rhythm is regular, because there will be fewer than three large squares between R waves.

A physical assessment is indicated because of the following: (1) Sinus tachycardia is a physiological response to other conditions, some of which may seriously compromise the patient's clinical course. (2) In the presence of acute ischemic changes, sinus tachycardia may trigger ventricular arrhythmias.

Fever, emotion, pain, and exercise can quickly be evaluated as possible causes. Some patients have an accelerated sinus rate because of a television program, visitors, or frightening or aggravating stimuli around them.

In the complete physical assessment of the patient, listen particularly for a third heart sound, since this, along with sinus tachycardia, is one of the first signs of congestive heart failure. Look for other signs of congestive heart failure.

If the sinus tachycardia is associated with dyspnea and sudden chest pain, pulmonary embolism should be suspected and the physician notified.

A 12-lead ECG should be run to ascertain the presence of infarct extension.

Variations

Sinus tachycardias vary only if they are part of a bradycardia-tachycardia syndrome or because of associated conditions, such as AV block, bundle-branch block, PVCs, or PACs.

The diagnosis of sinus tachycardia is made because of the underlying rhythm.

Differential Diagnosis

	Atrial tachycardia	Sinus tachycardia
P waves	Differ from sinus P	Same as sinus P
AV block	Usual	Unusual

	PSVT	Sinus tachycardia
Rate	>160 beats/min	<160 beats/min
P waves	Differ from sinus P	Same as sinus P
Vagal maneuver	Terminates	Slows momentarily

Treatment

None, although a clinical assessment is indicated and the cause of the sinus tachycardia is treated

Sinus Bradycardia

Sinus bradycardia is a regular sinus rhythm of less than 60 beats/min.

Pathophysiology and Mechanism

There is usually no pathology in sinus bradycardia unless it occurs as part of the sick sinus syndrome. It is either the normal response to decreased demand for blood flow, in which case the vagal stimulation is more and sympathetic stimulation less, resulting in decreased automaticity in the SA node, such as during sleep or in trained athletes, or it may be the result of increased vagal tone in myocardial infarction and may or may not be accompanied by hypotension.

ECG Characteristics

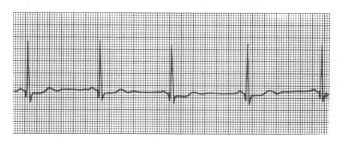

Rate: <60 beats/min

Rhythm: Regular

PR interval: Normal, although the PR may be too long or too short because of other conditions. All of the P waves are the same shape and are upright in leads I, II, aV_F, and V_4 to V_6.

QRS complex: Normal, although the QRS may be prolonged as a result of other conditions

Distinguishing features: Rate, rhythm, and uniform shape of the P waves

Causes

- Sleep
- Athletic heart
- Increased vagal tone
- Beta-adrenergic blockade

Nursing Implications

If the bradycardia is profound or there is AV dissociation, there may be hemodynamic compromise.

The slow rate is quickly diagnosed if the rhythm is regular, because there will be more than five large squares between R waves.

A physical assessment is indicated, because, although diastolic filling time is longer, the decrease in rate may compromise cardiac output. However, bradycardia is preferred to tachycardia in the setting of acute myocardial infarction.

Hemodynamic compromise is the only cause for concern or reason for intervention in this arrhythmia. Often the sinus rate will increase slightly if you converse with the patient or if the patient moves about.

If AV dissociation is present because of a junctional escape mechanism, there is no cause for concern unless the P wave is at the same time as or closely follows the QRS, in which case the atria are contracting against closed AV valves with resultant pressure backup into the pulmonary and systemic circulation.

Variations

Sinus bradycardias vary only if they are part of a bradycardia-tachycardia syndrome or because of associated conditions, such as AV block, bundle-branch block, PVCs, or PACs. The diagnosis of sinus bradycardia is made because of the underlying rhythm.

Differential Diagnosis

None

Treatment

Usually none, unless there is hemodynamic compromise and then IV atropine may be used

Sinus Arrhythmia

Sinus arrhythmia is an irregular sinus rhythm in which the cycle lengths vary so that the difference between the shortest PP interval and the longest PP interval is >0.12 sec.

Pathophysiology and Mechanism

There is no pathology in sinus arrhythmia. It is the normal response of the heart to respiration and is observed especially in children. The rate increases with inspiration and decreases with expiration. The vagus alternately causes increased and depressed automaticity secondary to respiration.

ECG Characteristics

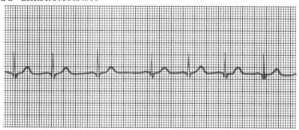

Rate: Varies with respiration—faster with inspiration—slower with expiration

Rhythm: Irregular

PR interval: Normal, although the PR may be too long or too short because of other conditions. All of the P waves are the same shape and are upright in leads I, II, aV_F, and V_4 to V_6.

QRS complex: Normal, although the QRS may be prolonged as a result of other conditions

Distinguishing features: Varying rate; cyclical, irregular rhythm; and uniform shape of the P waves

Cause

Normal respiratory pattern

Nursing Implications

The irregular rhythm and normal P waves help to diagnose this benign arrhythmia.

There may be hemodynamic compromise during the slower phase of this rhythm or because of AV dissociation as a result of junctional escape; often the sinus rate will increase slightly if you converse with the patient or have him move about in bed.

Variations

None

Differential Diagnosis

SA nodal reentry may resemble sinus arrhythmia, because the P waves are the same as normal sinus P waves in both rhythms. However, in SA reentry the transition to a faster rate is abrupt and not related to respiration.

Treatment

None

SA Block

SA block is a condition in which the sinus impulses are generated but not all of them are conducted, resulting in intermittently absent P waves.

Pathophysiology and Mechanism

There are conduction defects in the perinodal fibers.

ECG Characteristics

Rate: Normal, but varies because of pauses

Rhythm: Irregular

PR interval: Normal, although the PR may be too long or too short because of other conditions. All of the P waves are the same shape and upright in leads I, II, aV_F, and V_4 to V_6.

QRS complex: Normal, although the QRS may be prolonged as a result of other conditions.

Distinguishing features:

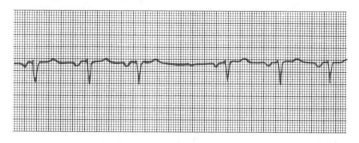

Type I (Wenckebach) SA block: PP intervals shorten until a P wave is dropped; pauses are less than twice the shortest cycle.

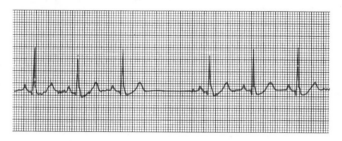

Type II SA block: PP intervals are an exact multiple of the sinus cycle and are regular before and after the dropped P wave.

Causes

- Digitalis, quinidine, or salicylates
- Coronary artery disease
- Acute infection
- Carotid sinus sensitivity and increased vagal tone

Nursing Implications

The diagnosis is made, after ruling out nonconducted PACs, because of pauses in the sinus rhythm.

There may be hemodynamic compromise if the pauses are too long.

The patient should be evaluated for decreased blood pressure, confusion, or increased number of ventricular ectopics, since these are the only reason for treating this arrhythmia.

The physician should be notified, because SA block is a possible manifestation of underlying heart disease, and a pacemaker may be indicated if there is hemodynamic compromise and the sinus node has not responded to treatment.

Variations

None

Differential Diagnosis

Nonconducted PACs are far more common and should be suspected first. Usually the P′ wave can be seen distorting the T wave before the pause. The diagnosis of sinus arrest can be made after ruling out nonconducted PACs and SA block.

Treatment

None, if there is no hemodynamic compromise. Otherwise IV atropine or a pacemaker may be indicated.

Sinus Arrest

Sinus arrest is a condition in which the sinus impulses are not generated, resulting in occasional absent P waves. If this condition is sustained, atrial standstill may result.

Pathophysiology and Mechanism

There is a marked depression in sinus node activity.

ECG Characteristics

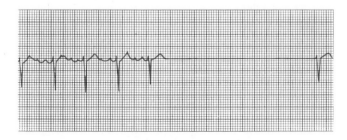

Rate: Normal, but varies because of pauses

Rhythm: Irregular

PR interval: Normal, although the PR may be too long or too short as a result of other conditions. All of the P waves are the same shape and are upright in leads I, II, aV_F, and V_4 to V_6.

QRS complex: Normal, although the QRS may be prolonged because of other conditions

Distinguishing features: Abrupt interruption of the sinus rhythm. PP interval of the pause is not a multiple of the sinus cycle

Causes

- Digitalis, quinidine, or salicylates
- Coronary artery disease
- Acute infection
- Carotid sinus sensitivity and increased vagal tone

Nursing Implications

The diagnosis is made, after ruling out nonconducted PACs, because of pauses in the sinus rhythm that are not multiples of the sinus rhythm.

There may be hemodynamic compromise if the pauses are too long.

The patient should be evaluated for decreased blood pressure, confusion, or increased number of ventricular ectopics, since these are the only reasons for treating this arrhythmia.

Variations

None

Differential Diagnosis

Nonconducted PACs are far more common and are always suspected first. Usually the P' wave can be seen distorting the T wave before the pause. The diagnosis of sinus arrest can be made after ruling out nonconducted PACs and SA block.

Treatment

None, if there is no hemodynamic compromise. Otherwise IV atropine or a pacemaker may be indicated.

Sick Sinus Syndrome

Sick sinus syndrome (SSS) is a combination of sinus node dysfunction and failure of an adequate escape pacemaker, resulting in cerebral dysfunction.

Pathophysiology and Mechanism

This syndrome may be either intrinsic or mediated by the autonomic nervous system. There may be a tendency to intranodal reentry, and there may be accessory pathways or inappropriate or absent sinus rhythms and failure of escape mechanisms.

ECG Characteristics

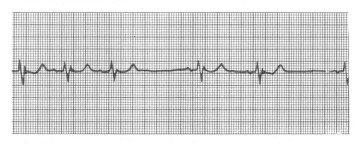

Rate: Too fast or too slow

Rhythm: Irregular

PR interval: May be abnormal

QRS complex: Normal, although the QRS may be prolonged because of other conditions

Distinguishing features: Any of the following arrhythmias may be present and associated with syncope:

Severe sinus bradycardia

Sinus arrest

Atrial standstill

SA block

Sinus bradycardia with recurring atrial fibrillation

Bradycardia-tachycardia

Temporary asystole following tachycardia or following electrical cardioversion of atrial tachyarrhythmia

Paroxysmal atrial fibrillation

Failure of the sinus node to accelerate in response to fever or exercise

Causes

- Ischemic disease
- Inflammatory diseases
- Amyloidosis
- Collagen disease
- Metastatic disease
- Surgical injury
- Idiopathic

Nursing Implications

The diagnosis is made because of the occurrence of a Stokes-Adams episode in association with supraventricular arrhythmias.

Take a careful history to see if there is a definable underlying cause, such as digitalis, beta blockers, calcium channel blockers, or (occasionally) diuretics.

Notify the physician and closely monitor the patient.

Be ready for emergency supportive measures. The patient may be a candidate for a permanent pacemaker and may require temporary emergency pacing if there is hemodynamic compromise and the sinus node has not responded to treatment.

Variations

There are many variations, among which are:

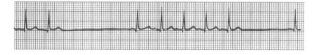

SSS with Type II second-degree SA block

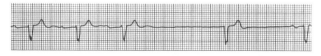

SSS in the form of a bradycardia-tachycardia syndrome

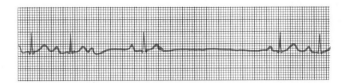

SSS with inappropriate overdrive suppression following an early PAC (in the T wave before the pause)

Differential Diagnosis

None

Treatment

Before a pacemaker is inserted, ensure that no drugs have been given at all for several days; the arrhythmia may be drug related.

Treatment of SSS is highly individualized.

Paroxysmal Sinus Tachycardia Resulting From SA Nodal Reentry

Paroxysmal sinus tachycardia is the sudden onset of sinus tachycardia.

Pathophysiology and Mechanism

There may or may not be pathology, since the SA node itself is the perfect type of tissue to support a reentry circuit. This can be initiated by a sinus impulse that does not exit the sinus node uniformly, leaving a nonrefractory pathway by which the impulse can return into the SA node and establish a reentry circuit.

ECG Characteristics

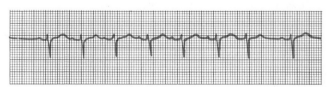

Rate: Too fast

Rhythm: Irregular

PR interval: Normal, although the PR may be too long or too short because of other conditions. All of the P waves are the same shape and are upright in leads I, II, aV_F, and V_4 to V_6.

QRS complex: Normal, although the QRS may be prolonged as a result of other conditions

Distinguishing Features:

Heart rate suddenly accelerates; tachycardia ends abruptly

Rhythm of the tachycardia usually regular

Normal sinus P waves

Causes

- Ischemia
- Cardiomyopathy

Nursing Implications

Usually none, unless there is acute myocardial infarction and then there may be hemodynamic compromise because of the tachycardia

Variations

None

Differential Diagnosis

Sinus arrhythmia

Treatment

None

Supraventricular Ectopics

3

PAC
Atrial flutter
Atrial fibrillation
Atrial tachycardia

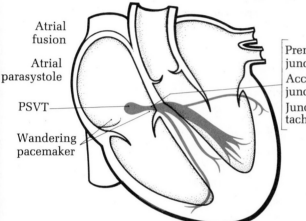

Atrial
fusion

Atrial
parasystole

PSVT

Wandering
pacemaker

Premature
junctional beat

Accelerated
junctional rhythm

Junctional
tachycardia

Supraventricular ectopic complexes and rhythms originate out-side the sinus node and above the branching portion of the bun-dle of His. They may be either abnormal premature mechanisms or normal escape mechanisms occuring in response to an abnor-mality in the sinus node. The two most common mechanisms involved are enhanced automaticity in the atria or AV junc-tion (bundle of His) and AV nodal reentry or reentry using an accessory pathway (WPW syndrome). The arrhythmias asso-ciated with WPW syndrome are discussed in Chapter 9.

Enhanced automaticity may be secondary to digitalis tox-icity, electrolyte imbalance, hypoxia, myocardial stretch, or acute myocardial infarction and may result in single PACs or PJCs, ectopic atrial tachycardia, accelerated junctional rhythm, or junctional tachycardia.

An AV nodal reentry mechanism may be initiated by a single premature atrial, junctional, or ventricular complex, resulting in paroxysmal supraventricular tachycardia (PSVT).

Anatomy and Physiology

Atrial ectopic foci are located within the atria and are the result of enhanced automaticity or afterdepolarizations. They may produce isolated or frequent PACs or atrial tachycardia and may precipitate atrial fibrillation or flutter.

Junctional ectopic foci are located in the bundle of His and are also the result of enhanced automaticity. They may produce isolated or frequent PJCs or an accelerated junctional or idiojunctional rhythm that may be fast enough to qualify as a junctional tachycardia.

The PACs or PJCs may precipitate an AV nodal reentry mechanism located within the AV node proper or an AV reentry mechanism involving the AV node and an accessory pathway, and result in PSVT.

Atrial Ectopic Mechanisms
Premature Atrial Complexes

PACs are premature atrial beats that originate outside of the sinus node. The resulting ECG deflection is called a P' (P prime) wave.

Pathophysiology and Mechanism

PACs are a result of enhanced automaticity or afterdepolarizations. The mechanisms of AV conduction and compensatory pauses following PACs are described here.

AV conduction. The PAC may be so premature that it is not conducted at all, because both bundle branches are refractory; or it may be conducted down only one bundle branch, and be blocked in the other (aberrant ventricular conduction).

Less-than-full compensatory pause. The PAC resets the SA node, causing the next expected sinus P wave to be on time *if measured from the PAC,* but earlier than it would have been if the sinus node had not been disturbed.

Full or more-than-full compensatory pause. The PAC may suppress the SA node (overdrive suppression) and cause the next few sinus cycles to lengthen.

ECG Characteristics

PAC

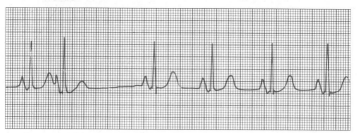

Rate: that of the underlying rhythm

Rhythm: Irregular, resulting from PACs (underlying rhythm may be regular)

PR interval: Normal, although the PR interval may be too long or too short because of other conditions. All of the P waves are the same shape and upright in leads I, II, aV$_F$, and V$_4$ to V$_6$.

[The P'-R interval may be the same, longer, or shorter than the PR interval, or the P' wave may not be conducted to the ventricles (a blocked PAC).]

QRS complex: Normal, although the QRS may be prolonged as a result of aberrancy or other conditions

Distinguishing features: Normal QRS and a P' wave that is premature and different in shape from the sinus P wave

Causes

- Various stimuli—emotion, tobacco, or coffee
- Congestive heart failure (in the setting of myocardial infarction)
- Atrial dilation or hypertrophy resulting from mitral stenosis or atrial septal defect
- Electrolyte imbalance
- Hypoxia
- Digitalis toxicity

Nursing Implications

In the setting of acute myocardial infarction, PACs are frequently a result of the catecholamines released secondary to apprehension and pain. Once the patient is reassured and given morphine the PACs often disappear. Also, since many people still smoke and come in with hypoxia (a cause of atrial ectopy), oxygen will effectively treat the PACs.

The diagnosis is made because of an irregular rhythm and premature, ectopic-looking P waves, which may be clearly visible or may distort T waves.

Although PACs are not life threatening, in association with acute myocardial infarction they warn of congestive heart failure and/or electrolyte imbalance. PACs, along with sinus tachycardia and a third heart sound, are early signs of congestive heart failure.

PACs may precipitate a rapid ventricular rate secondary to atrial flutter, fibrillation, or PSVT. The resulting fall in cardiac output may cause further myocardial damage and may precipitate ventricular tachycardia. Thus possible causes should be identified and treated.

If bigeminal nonconducted PACs develop, the resulting bradycardia may be profound and may cause hemodynamic deterioration, even in the otherwise healthy heart.

Variations

PAC   PAC

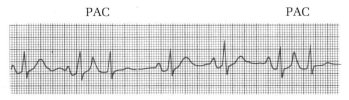

PACs hidden in T waves

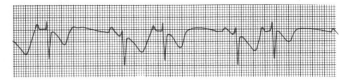

Bigeminal PACs

PAC

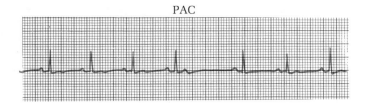

Nonconducted PACs

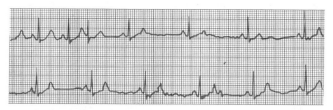

Bigeminal nonconducted PACs

Differential Diagnosis

Sinus arrest or SA block. Nonconducted PACs are statistically far more common and can usually be spotted distorting the T wave.

Treatment

PACs are not treated, but in association with acute myocardial infarction, their cause is identified and treated.

Atrial Tachycardia

Atrial tachycardia is an ectopic atrial rhythm with a rate of 140 to 250 beats/min.

Pathophysiology and Mechanism

Atrial tachycardia is a result of enhanced automaticity and may be seen with any type of heart disease. When there is a rapidly firing atrial ectopic stimulus, the normal response of the AV node is to block; the faster the atrial rate, the more severe the AV block.

ECG Characteristics

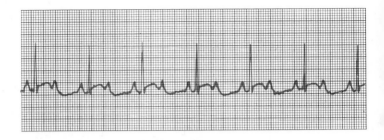

Rate: 140 to 250 beats/min (atrial). The ventricular rate depends on the AV conduction ratio.

Rhythm: Regular

PR interval: Not applicable; P'-R interval may be normal or prolonged. The P waves are ectopic.

QRS complex: Normal, although the QRS may be prolonged because of other conditions.

Distinguishing features: Rate and AV conduction ratio, which is usually 2:1. In digitalis toxicity the P wave axis is often superior-inferior (positive in inferior leads), and often in 2:1 block the PP interval across the QRS is shorter than the one without a QRS (ventriculo-phasic PP interval).

Causes

- Digitalis toxicity
- Heart disease

Nursing Implications

The diagnosis is made because of a rapid, regular atrial rhythm that is not interrupted by a vagal maneuver. There is usually a 2:1 AV conduction ratio.

Atrial tachycardia may be a sign of digitalis toxicity.

Atrial tachycardia may deteriorate into atrial flutter or fibrillation. The resulting fall in cardiac output may cause further myocardial damage and may precipitate ventricular tachycardia. Thus an attempt should be made to identify and treat the cause of the atrial tachycardia.

Variations

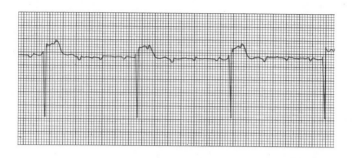

Atrial tachycardia with 4:1 AV conduction (other conduction ratios are also possible)

Differential Diagnosis

	Atrial Ectopic Tachycardia	PSVT (AV nodal reentry)	Sinus Tachycardia
P waves	Visible	Usually buried within QRS complex; may distort V_1 patterns (pseudo RBBB)	Visible
	+ in II, III, and aV_F (digitalis toxicity)	Retrograde (negative in II, III, and aV_F)	Normal
Rate	Gradually increases ("warm-up")	Begins abruptly and remains same; ends abruptly	Gradually increases; gradually decreases
P'-R interval	Normal	Long (first one)	Normal

Treatment

Identify and treat the cause.

Chaotic Atrial Tachycardia

Chaotic atrial tachycardia is a multifocal atrial tachycardia.

ECG Characteristics

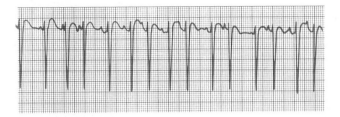

Rate: 100 to 250 beats/min
Rhythm: Irregular
PR interval: May or may not be normal. P'-R intervals may vary.
QRS complex: Normal
Distinguishing features: P' waves of several different shapes and an irregular rhythm

Pathophysiology and Mechanism

Multifocal areas of enhanced automaticity or afterdepolarizations, usually secondary to chronic lung disease.

Causes

- Chronic pulmonary disease
- Hypoxia
- Electrolyte derangement

Nursing Implications

This arrhythmia carries a high mortality and all of the nursing implications of the primary disease.

Variations

None

Differential Diagnosis

Atrial fibrillation

Treatment

Chaotic atrial tachycardia is a difficult arrhythmia to treat; it is more often seen in the respiratory unit than in the CCU.

Atrial Flutter

Atrial flutter is a rapid atrial ectopic tachycardia of two types.

Pathophysiology and Mechanism

The mechanism of type I atrial flutter is a reentry circuit within the right atrium; the mechanism of type II is not known.

AV conduction is usually 2:1, 4:1, 6:1, and so on (in even numbers). Wenckebach conduction is often the case at the lower level of the AV node, with 2:1 at the top of the AV node. Thus every other beat that is conducted through the top of the AV node is then conducted with lengthening conduction times until a beat is dropped. This results in group beating of the ventricular rhythm.

ECG Characteristics

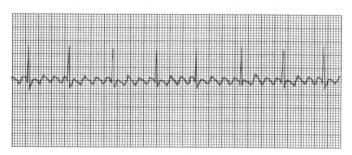

Rate: In type I (classical) the atrial rate ranges from 230-350 beats/min; in type II the range is 340-430 beats/min.

Rhythm: Atrial rhythm is regular; ventricular rhythm depends on the AV conduction pattern.

P'-R interval: 0.26 to 0.46 sec

QRS complex: Normal

Distinguishing features:

Regular sawtooth pattern in II, III, aVF

Sharp positive P' waves in V_1

Normal QRS complexes

AV conduction in 2:1 to 8:1 ratios
T wave may distort the flutter pattern.

Causes

- Any form of heart disease
- Acute illness

Nursing Implications

Atrial flutter is rarely seen in normal hearts and is more common in patients over 40 years of age with myocardial ischemia.

Be sure that the patient has enough oxygen.

If the onset is sudden, notify the physician and prepare to digitalize the patient or perform cardioversion.

Variations

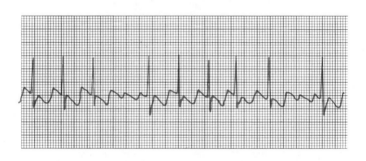

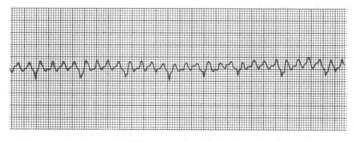

Varying degrees of AV conduction ratios

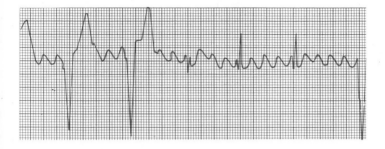

Atrial flutter with AV dissociation (an accelerated idioventricular rhythm).

Differential Diagnosis

When the conduction ratio is 2:1, atrial flutter is often mistaken for sinus tachycardia of 140 to 175 beats/min. The ventricular rate makes one suspicious of a hidden flutter wave, and usually the onset of the R wave is distorted by the flutter wave.

Treatment

Atrial flutter is usually managed by cardioversion, pharmacological or electrical, since the ventricular response is not as easy to control pharmacologically as is that in atrial fibrillation. Type I atrial flutter can be converted with rapid atrial pacing. However, type II often requires aggressive pharmacological treatment to slow the rapid ventricular rate.

 # Atrial Fibrillation

Atrial fibrillation is an ectopic atrial arrhythmia characterized by erratic depolarization of the atria.

Pathophysiology and Mechanism

In atrial fibrillation the atria are quivering chambers connecting the ventricles with the great vessels. There is no organized atrial contraction, the atrial kick is lost, and cardiac output decreases. In untreated atrial fibrillation the ventricular rate is usually rapid, decreasing cardiac output further, resulting in congestive heart failure, hypotension, possibly cardiogenic shock, and myocardial ischemia. The inefficient movement of blood in the atria predisposes the patient to the formation of emboli. The mechanism of atrial fibrillation is not known.

ECG Characteristics

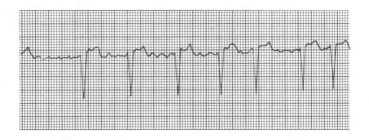

Rate: Uncontrolled, 110 to 180 beats/min; controlled, 70 to 80 beats/min

Rhythm: Irregular

PR interval: Absent P waves

QRS complex: Normal

Distinguishing features: Absent P waves and irregular ventricular response

Causes

- Mitral disease
- Ischemic disease
- Hypertension
- Thyrotoxicosis
- Increasing left-atrial size in elderly patients

Nursing Implications

The diagnosis is made by the absent P waves and an irregular ventricular rhythm.

If the onset is sudden, the hemodynamic consequences of a sudden drop in cardiac output may be profound, and the physician should be notified. Prepare for cardioversion and evaluate for shock and myocardial ischemia (anginal chest pain, ST segment depressions of elevations, new Q waves, (inverted T waves).

If the arrhythmia is chronic, evaluate for:

1. Digitalis toxicity, if applicable (QRS regularity, group beating, ventricular ectopics, or symptoms, such as visual complaints, restlessness, agitation, drowsiness, loss of memory, weakness, and fatigue; neurolgic pain in lumbar region, teeth, mandible, or maxila; and abdominal pain, diarrhea, and vomiting)
2. Congestive heart failure (difficult breathing, pedal edema, and crackles at lung bases)

Variations

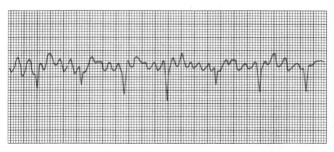

Coarse atrial fibrillation with signs of digitalis toxicity (regularization of the ventricular response)

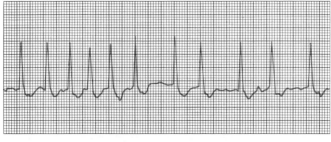

Fine atrial fibrillation with uncontrolled ventricular response

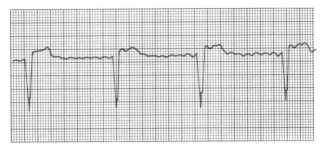

Atrial fibrillation with complete AV block

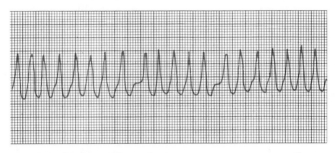

Atrial fibrillation with conduction over an accessory pathway

Differential Diagnosis

None

Treatment

In the setting of acute myocardial infarction, atrial fibrillation is an ominous rhythm, since there are no atrial contractions that can participate in ventricular filling. Also, the changing cycle length results in many cycles with a short diastolic filling time and demands that there be an increase in left-atrial pressure to achieve filling during the short diastolic interludes. Cardioversion is therefore the treatment of choice in this clinical setting. If, however, the rhythm is well tolerated, digitalis or verapamil may be the treatment of choice, but with awareness of the effects of verapamil on the peripheral vasculature.

Chronic atrial fibrillation may not convert to normal sinus

rhythm with therapy, and, since the purpose of treatment for these patients is to control the ventricular response and thus improve cardiac output, digitalis or verapamil is often used. In atrial fibrillation of recent onset, there is a possibility that the arrhythmia can be converted with drugs or electrical cardioversion.

Wandering Pacemaker

A wandering pacemaker is an atrial or junctional ectopic rhythm that has approximately the same rate as the sinus node and therefore competes for control of the heart. If the term must be used at all, it is best reserved for sinus slowing with an escape pacemaker. In this context it is usually in a normal heart; in association with myocardial infarction, it occurs because of vagotonia.

Pathophysiology and Mechanism

The ectopic pacemaker competes with the sinus rhythm because it is approximately the same rate. It is clear then that the wandering pacemaker may be either a passive escape mechanism or an active intruder; thus the term is merely descriptive and not a primary diagnosis.

ECG Characteristics

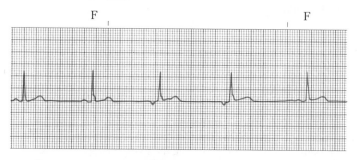

Rate: Normal or < 60 min
Rhythm: Slightly irregular
PR interval: Normal
QRS complex: Normal
Distinguishing features: A sinus rhythm that gives way to

an ectopic atrial or junctional rhythm, often with atrial fusion beats at the transitions; there is retrograde conduction to the atria from the junctional focus

Causes

- Sinus bradycardia
- Accelerated atrial or junctional rhythm secondary to digitalis toxicity

Nursing Implications

The wandering pacemaker, when noted, should not be offered as a diagnosis, since it is merely a descriptive term. The ectopic rhythm could be a normal escape mechanism or an enhanced ectopic rhythm.

Determine the rate of the ectopic rhythm and that of the sinus node. If the ectopic rhythm is less than 60 beats/min, it is most probably a normal escape mechanism and the only concern is the hemodynamic status of the patient. However, if the ectopic rhythm is more than 60 beats/min, an accelerated ectopic focus is present, and a clinical assessment is indicated to determine the cause even though the heart rate is within "normal" limits and the patient is hemodynamically stable.

Variations

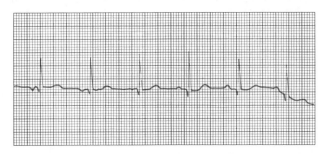

Normal sinus rhythm with an accelerated junctional or atrial rhythm

Differential Diagnosis

None

Treatment

If there is a normal escape mechanism, no treatment is indicated unless there is hemodynamic deterioration and then IV atropine may be appropriate. Ask the patient to cough; coughing decreases vagal tone and promotes the reappearance of the sinus rhythm if it is available. If the ectopic rhythm is enhanced then the cause should be sought and treated.

Junctional Ectopic Mechanisms

Premature and Escape Junctional Beats

A junctional beat originates in the bundle of His, may be either premature or escape, and may or may not have retrograde conduction to the atria.

Pathophysiology and Mechanism

Premature junctional complexes (PJC) are a result of enhanced automaticity in the bundle of His, which may be secondary to digitalis toxicity. When the ectopic focus discharges, the current may or many not be blocked in the retrograde direction into the atria. If retrograde conduction is not blocked there will be a retrograde P′ wave that may be before, during (not seen), or after the QRS complex, depending on the relative speeds of anterograde and retrograde conduction and the location of the ectopic focus in the bundle of His. Whether or not there is retrograde conduction does not change the clinical implications of the arrhythmia.

Escape junctional beats are a normal mechanism designed to protect the ventricles from excessively slow rates when the sinus node is too slow or AV conduction fails.

ECG Characteristics

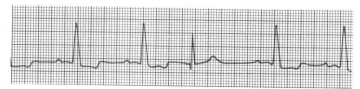

Rate: That of the underlying rhythm

Rhythm: Irregular as a result of the PJCs (underlying rhythm may be regular)

PR interval: Normal in the underlying sinus rhythm. The P′ wave associated with the junctional beat may be absent if there is no retrograde conduction to the atria; if present, it is negative in II, III, and a V_F, and may appear before, during, or after the QRS complex.

QRS complex: Normal, although the QRS may be prolonged as a result of other conditions.

Distinguishing features: Normal QRS complex and a P′ wave that is not seen, buried in the QRS complex, or negative in II, III, and aV_F. If the P′ wave precedes the QRS it does so by no more than 0.12 sec.

Causes

Premature junctional complexes may be caused by the following:
- Digitalis
- Acute inferior-wall myocardial infarction
- Tricuspid prosthesis
- Rheumatic fever

Escape junctional beats are caused by excessively long pauses in the cardiac cycle.

Nursing Implications

In the setting of acute myocardial infarction, a physical assessment is indicated for the purpose of defining the cause of the junctional enhanced automaticity, or, in the case of junctional escape beats, assessing the hemodynamic effect of the bradycardia.

The diagnosis is made because of normal-looking QRS complexes that may be associated with a retrograde P′ wave (negative in II, III, and aV_F).

If the patient is taking digitalis, premature junctional beats should be regarded as one of the first signs of digitalis toxicity.

The physician should be notified. Digitalis levels and electrolyte levels may be ordered.

With bradycardia and/or AV block the hemodynamic condition of the patient will dictate the appropriate nursing response. If there is hemodynamic deterioration, the physician should be notified; IV atropine or a pacemaker may be indicated.

Variations

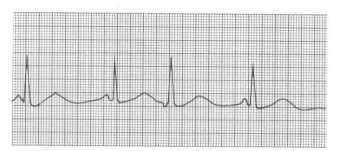

PJC with the P′ preceding the QRS complex

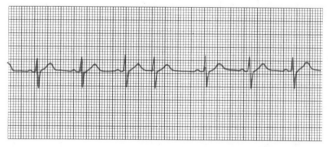

PJC with the P′ hidden in the QRS complex

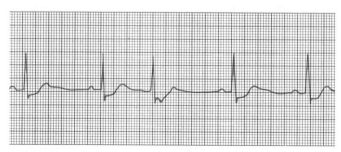

PJC with the P′ following the QRS complex

Differential Diagnosis

None

Treatment

PJCs are not treated, but their cause is identified and treated.

Accelerated Idiojunctional Rhythm

An accelerated idiojunctional rhythm is an ectopic rhythm located in the bundle of His and controlling the ventricles at a rate of 60 to 100 beats/min. When the rate exceeds 100 beats/min, it is termed junctional tachycardia.

Pathophysiology and Mechanism

Enhanced automaticity in the bundle of His, which may be secondary to digitalis toxicity

ECG Characteristics

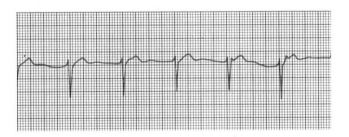

Rate: 60 to 100 beats/min

Rhythm: Regular

PR interval: Normal in the underlying sinus rhythm. When the junctional focus begins to take over, the PR interval may appear to shorten; however, when this happens there is no relationship between the P wave and QRS complex (AV dissociation).

QRS complex: Normal, although the QRS complex may be prolonged as a result of other conditions

Distinguishing features: A junctional rhythm reveals itself when its rate is about the same as that of the sinus node, resulting in AV dissociation. The P waves get closer and closer to the QRS complex as the rate of the junctional focus exceeds that of the sinus node.

Causes

- Myocardial infarction
- Digitalis toxicity

Nursing Implications

A physical assessment is indicated for the purpose of defining the cause of the junctional ectopy.

The diagnosis is made on the basis of a junctional rhythm taking over from the sinus rhythm and resulting in AV dissociation.

If the patient is taking digitalis, this rhythm should be regarded as one of the first signs of digitalis toxicity.

The physician should be notified; digitalis levels and electrolyte levels may be ordered.

During the periods of AV dissociation there may be hemodynamic deterioration. In the setting of acute myocardial infarction this may cause the area of injury and ischemia to extend.

Variations

None

Differential Diagnosis

None

Treatment

Identify and treat the cause.

Junctional Tachycardia

Junctional tachycardia is an ectopic rhythm resulting from a focus of enhanced automaticity located in the bundle of His and controlling the ventricles at a rate of 100 to 130 beats/min. If the rate is less than 100 beats/min, it is termed accelerated junctional or idiojunctional rhythm.

Pathophysiology and Mechanism

Enhanced automaticity in the bundle of His, which may be secondary to digitalis toxicity, is present. The junctional ectopic focus paces the ventricles, and there may or may not be retrograde conduction to the atria. If there is not retrograde conduction, then there is AV dissociation. If there is retrograde conduction, then the hemodynamic situation may also be serious, since the P′ wave may coincide with or follow the QRS complex, causing the atria to contract against closed AV valves and forcing a backup pressure into the systemic and pulmonary circulations.

ECG Characteristics

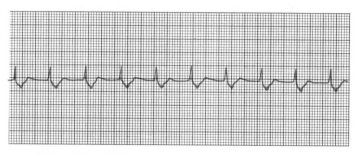

Rate: 100 to 130 beats/min

Rhythm: Regular

PR interval: Not applicable. P′-R interval: When the junctional focus begins to take over, the PR interval may appear to shorten; however, when this happens there is no relationship between the P and the QRS complex (AV dissociation). The P′ will be absent if there is no retrograde conduction to the atria; if present, it is negative in II, III, and aV$_F$ and may be before, during, or after the QRS complex, depending on the relative speeds of anterograde and retrograde conduction and the location of the ectopic focus in the bundle of His.

QRS complex: Normal, although the QRS complex may be prolonged as a result of other conditions

Distinguishing features: A junctional rhythm of more than 100 beats/min. The QRS complex will be narrow if there is no associated intraventricular conduction problem.

Causes

- Myocardial infarction
- Digitalis toxicity

Nursing Implications

A physical assessment is indicated for the purpose of defining the cause of the junctional ectopy.

Warning arrhythmias are PJCs and accelerated junctional rhythm.

The diagnosis is made when there is a junctional rhythm at a rate greater than 100 beats/min.

If the patient is taking digitalis, this rhythm should be regarded as one of the later signs of digitalis toxicity.

The physician should be notified; digitalis levels and electrolyte levels may be ordered.

Variations

None

Differential Diagnosis

If the mechanism is understood, there is usually no differential diagnosis unless the junctional tachycardia exceeds 130 beats/min and then there may be difficulty in differentiating it from an AV nodal reentry mechanism (PSVT). A vagal maneuver usually interrupts the PSVT and has no effect on junctional tachycardia.

Treatment

Identify and treat the cause

Paroxysmal Supraventricular Tachycardia Resulting From AV Nodal Reentry

Paroxysmal supraventricular tachycardia (PSVT) begins and ends abruptly; it is supported by either an AV nodal reentry circuit (discussed here) or by an AV reentry circuit (an accessory pathway, discussed later) and achieves rates of 170 to 250 beats/min.

Pathophysiology and Mechanism

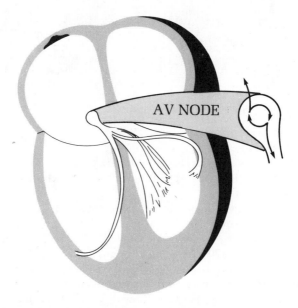

AV nodal reentry is possible because of the existence of two functionally separate pathways within the node, a slow (alpha) pathway and a fast (beta) pathway. The refractory period of the slow pathway is the shortest; therefore when an early atrial beat arrives, it may be conducted only down the slow pathway to the ventricles. By this time the fast pathway has recovered and the impulse returns by it to the atria. It is then conducted back down the slow pathway to reactivate the ventricles—and so on, around and around in the AV node.

ECG Characteristics

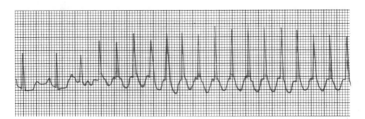

Rate: 170 to 250 beats/min

Rhythm: Regular

PR interval: Not applicable. May be normal in the sinus rhythm. The P'R interval at the onset of the tachycardia is abnormally long.

QRS complex: Similar to the sinus-conducted QRS complex; rarely aberrant

Distinguishing features: A narrow QRS tachycardia that usually exceeds 170 beats/min and begins abruptly with a prolonged P'R interval. This is necessary to accommodate the refractoriness and establish the reentry circuit. The rest of the P' waves will either not be seen or they will distort the end of the QRS (P' waves just barely showing). There is no alternans of the QRS after the first 5 to 6 seconds. May be interrupted by a vagal maneuver.

Causes

- One early PAC
- Rarely a PJC

Nursing Implications

The diagnosis is made because of a narrow QRS tachycardia that begins and ends abruptly. This rhythm must be differentiated from that of circus movement tachycardia using an accessory pathway. Before terminating the tachycardia, secure as many leads as possible, preferably I, II, III, V_1, and V_6. Look for P waves. In AV nodal reentry the P' waves are hidden within or peeking out at the end of the QRS. Observe for alternans (alternating QRS heights); after the first 5 to 6 seconds there is no alternans in AV nodal reentry.

Variations

Common: AV nodal reentry using a slow anterograde intranodal pathway and a fast retrograde pathway, causing simultaneous atrial and ventricular activation (P' buried within or peeking out at the end of the QRS).

Rare: AV nodal reentry using a fast anterograde intranodal pathway and a slow retrograde pathway, causing atrial activation to follow ventricular activation with a long RP interval (RP > PR).

Differential Diagnosis

	Atrial Ectopic Tachycardia	PSVT (AV nodal reentry)	Sinus Tachycardia
P waves	Visible	Usually buried within QRS complex; may distort V_1 patterns (pseudo RBBB)	Visible
	+ or − in II, III, and aV_F	Retrograde (negative in II, III, and aV_F)	Normal
Rate	Gradually increases ("warm-up")	Begins abruptly and remains same; ends abruptly	Gradually increases; gradually decreases
P'-R interval	Normal	Long (first one)	Normal

Treatment

1. Use vagal maneuver first.
2. If vagal maneuver is unsuccessful, the treatment that follows depends on the patients' hemodynamic status. Procainamide (or propranolol) or DC cardioversion may be used. Although verapamil and propranolol block the AV node, they also lower the blood pressure, and this must be considered. Digitalis shortens the refractory period of an accessory pathway and is avoided if an accessory pathway is suspected to exist.

Vagotonic Maneuvers for PSVT

Carotid sinus stimulation

Rationale. The carotid sinus is located at the angle of the jaw (not in the neck). Of the vagotonic maneuvers, carotid sinus stimulation is a good one if done by health professionals. The purpose is to create an elevation of blood pressure in the carotid sinus so that there will be reflex slowing of AV conduction. This is achieved by pressing the carotid sinus against the lateral processes of the vertebra. Such a manuever will cause pain, and the patient should be warned of this and told that it will last for only a few seconds.

Technique. Grip the patient's chin with your right palm and swing your right thumb around; you will find that it automatically falls at the angle of the jaw, the location of the carotid bifurcation. You can now press rather forcefully with the thumb for not more than 3 seconds—pressure for any longer may be dangerous.

Precautions. Be sure that you have already listened for carotid bruits and have taken a history regarding any transient ischemic attacks. Never perform carotid sinus stimulation without ECG monitoring so that the results can be observed and responded to if necessary. The carotid sinus maneuver is relatively safe and effective.

Gagging: This is a good vagotonic manuever. If the episodes of PSVT occur, instruct the patient to try to vomit,

Trendelenburg position: The patient can be instructed to do this at home.

Valsalva maneuver: Blowing against a closed glottis is an effective vagotonic maneuver.

Squatting: For the young patient, "hunkering down" (squatting with hands gripped across the belly and pulling in) is a fairly easy thing to do and is very effective. This is obviously not for the older patient who can't squat.

NOTE: Eyeball pressure is not only ineffective, but *it is dangerous;* cases of retinal detachment have been reported.

Atrial Fusion Complexes

An atrial fusion complex is the complex that results when two impulses collide within the atria.

Pathophysiology and Mechanism

Atrial fusion beats result from the presence of two opposing electrical currents (sinus and atrial ectopic) within the same chamber at the same time. The resultant P wave is often narrower and of lesser amplitude than the P′ wave alone. Atrial fusion is seen in association with atrial parasystole and wandering pacemaker.

ECG Characteristics

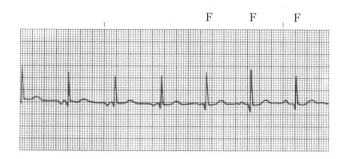

Rate: That of the underlying rhythm
Rhythm: Regular
PR interval: The PR interval of the fusion beat is the same as that of the sinus rhythm. The P wave of the fusion beat is sometimes isoelectric or intermediate between the P waves of the fusing impulses.
QRS complex: That of the underlying rhythm.
Distinguishing features: There are other atrial ectopic beats in the tracing, and there is reason to believe that one was due at the same time as the sinus P wave.

Causes

- That of the atrial ectopic beat or rhythm

Nursing Implications

Atrial fusion beats may be the result of a passive escape mechanism or an active intruder. If the rate of the atrial ectopic rhythm takes over from an adequate sinus rhythm of 58 to 60 beats/min, a clinical assessment is indicated to determine the cause of the atrial ectopy. If the sinus rhythm is too slow and the atrial ectopic rhythm is a protective escape mechanism, the prime consideration is hemodynamics. If there is hemodynamic deterioration, the sinus rate should be increased.

Variations

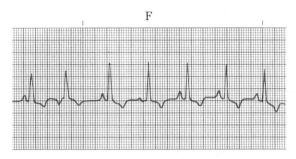

F

Atrial parasystole

Wandering pacemaker

Differential Diagnosis

None

Treatment

Usually none

Atrial Parasystole

Atrial parasystole is an independent and undisturbable ectopic rhythm whose pacemaker cannot be discharged by impulses of the dominant (usually sinus) rhythm. It is far less common than ventricular parasystole.

Pathophysiology and Mechanism

Atrial parasystole occurs when an area of enhanced automaticity in the atria is encircled by tissue that is so depressed that the ectopic impulses can exit across it but the sinus impulse cannot enter to discharge it.

ECG Characteristics

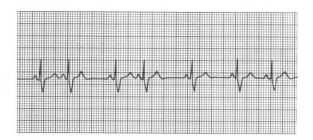

Rate: That of the underlying rhythm
Rhythm: Irregular, because of atrial premature beats
PR interval: Normal
QRS complex: Normal
Distinguishing features:
Atrial ectopics with no fixed coupling
Interectopic intervals that are multiples of a common denominator
Fusion beats

Cause

- Myocardial infarction

Nursing Implications

This is a benign arrhythmia.

Variations

None

Differential Diagnosis

PACs

Treatment

Usually none

Ventricular Ectopics

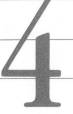

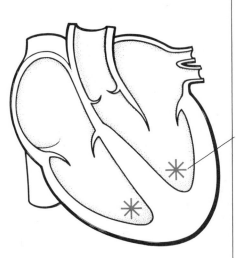

- PVC
- Ventricular tachycardia
- Ventricular fibrillation
- Torsades de pointes
- Accelerated idioventricular rhythm
- Ventricular parasystole
- Ventricular fusion
- Ventricular flutter
- Ventricular escape

Ventricular ectopics are the result of enhanced automaticity, reentry, or afterdepolarizations and take the form of premature beats, ventricular tachycardia, ventricular fibrillation, accelerated idioventricular rhythm, or parasystole. Premature ventricular complexes (PVCs) may be right or left ventricular, unifocal, multifocal, bigeminal, interpolated, R-on-T, end-diastolic, or fusion beats; in the setting of acute myocardial infarction, they are considered dangerous and are aggressively treated.

Premature Ventricular Complexes

PVCs are premature ectopic beats originating in the ventricles (below the branching of the bundle of His).

Pathophysiology and Mechanism

Either there is an area of enhanced automaticity in the ventricles or there are afterdepolarizations or reentry circuits. The reentry circuits are usually microreentry, involving a microscopic amount of His-Purkinje tissue. A macroreentry circuit is also possible, involving the bundle branches and the bundle of His. PVCs may be the result of myocardial infarction or ischemia without infarction or may occur from unknown causes in otherwise healthy hearts.

The full compensatory pause. If the PVC does not have retrograde conduction to the atria (Fig. 4-1), the sinus rhythm will not be interrupted, although the sinus P wave close to the PVC will not be conducted. In this case, you should be able to walk out the P waves across the PVC. The pause resulting from the nonconducted sinus P wave is called a full compensatory pause.

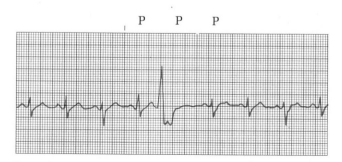

Figure 4-1
Full compensatory pause. Note that all sinus P waves can be seen.

ECG Characteristics

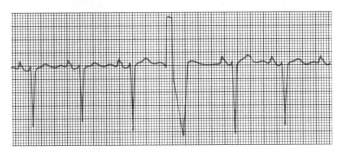

Rate: That of the underlying rhythm

Rhythm: Irregular, because of PVC

PR interval: That of the underlying rhythm; there is no P wave associated with the PVC

QRS complex: That of the PVC is broad; that of the underlying rhythm may be normal

Distinguishing features: No related P wave; premature, broad QRS complex; T wave of opposite polarity

Causes

- Catecholamines
- Caffeine
- Drugs (epinephrine, isoproterenol, or aminophylline)
- Digitalis
- Hypokalemia
- Hypomagnesemia
- Hypoxia
- Ischemia
- Myocardial infarction
- Significant anemia
- Myocardial stretch

Nursing Implications

A diagnosis is made because of premature, broad QRS complexes with no associated P or P′ wave.

In heart disease or after myocardial infarction, PVCs are common and are associated with an increased incidence of ventricular tachycardia, ventricular fibrillation, and sudden death. Therefore in this clinical setting they are aggressively treated, especially if they are paired, multifocal, or R-on-T.

In individuals with apparently normal hearts, PVCs are not associated with an increased risk of sudden death and are not treated.

Variations

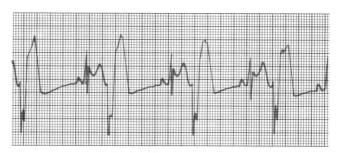

Unifocal PVCs and ventricular bigeminy

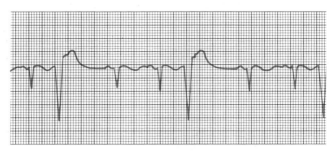

Ventricular trigeminy (two normal and one PVC)

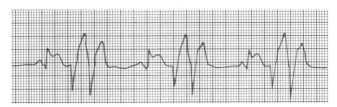

Ventricular trigeminy (one normal and two PVCs)

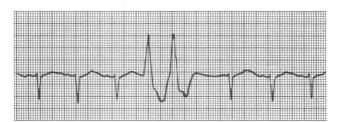

Paired PVCs

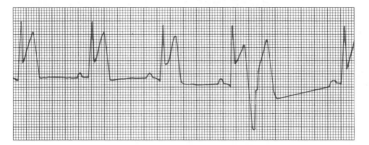

R-on-T phenomenon

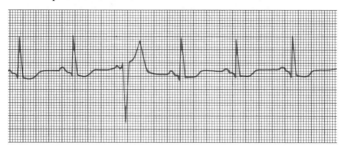

End-diastolic PVC

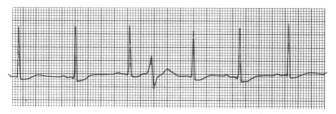

Interpolated PVC

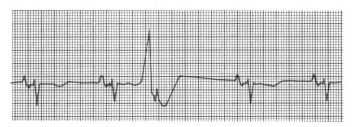

PVC with retrograde conduction to the atria

V_1

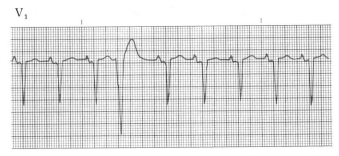

Right-ventricular PVC

V_1

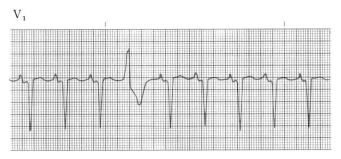

Left-ventricular PVC

Differential Diagnosis

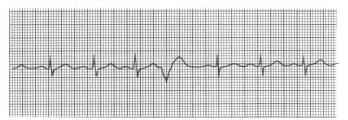

PAC with aberrant ventricular conduction

Unless a P′ wave can be seen in front of the broad beat (as in this case, distorting the T) or you have morphological proof of ventricular aberrancy, a diagnosis of ventricular ectopy should be made.

Treatment

In the diseased, ischemic, or infarcted heart, antiarrhythmics (lidocaine or procainamide) are given.

 Ventricular Tachycardia

Ventricular tachycardia (VT) is an ectopic ventricular rhythm with a rate of 100 to 170 beats/min.

Pathophysiology and Mechanism

Ventricular tachycardia is most often thought to be the result of a microreentry circuit within the ventricles. Enhanced automaticity and afterdepolarizations are other causes.

ECG Characteristics

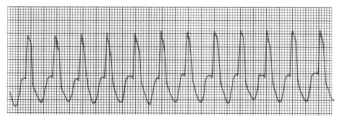

Rate: 100 to 170 beats/min
Rhythm: Regular 75% of the time

PR interval: Not applicable

QRS complex: > 0.12 sec and most often > 0.14 sec

Distinguishing features: Broad QRS complex with a regular rhythm and a rate between 100 and 170 beats/min. Left axis deviation, and in V_1 a monophasic R, QR, qR, RS, or a "rabbit ear" configuration (that is, two peaks, the first being the tallest). In slower rates, AV dissociation may be seen; however, 40% have retrograde conduction to the atria.

Causes (Incomplete List)

- Significant underlying cardiac disease
- Acute myocardial infarction
- Coronary artery disease
- Drugs (digitalis, isoproterenol)
- May occur in absence of evidence of structural heart disease

Nursing Implications

The diagnosis is made because of a broad QRS (> 0.12 sec) tachycardia that is often regular and has a rate of less than 170 beats/min. Left axis deviation and typical morphology in V_1 and V_6 and AV dissociation may be noted.

Ventricular tachycardia is life threatening and may deteriorate into ventricular fibrillation.

The chest thump is only rarely successful and is not recommended as a general rule. However, if you have observed the onset of ventricular tachycardia, give the patient a sharp thump to the midsternum with your clenched fist. This will deliver about 5 mV to the heart, and, if administered early, this may be enough to interrupt a reentry circuit. Have a defibrillator at hand, since the chest thump can potentially increase the rate of the ventricular tachycardia and precipitate ventricular fibrillation.

If this does not work, synchronized DC countershock is indicated; 10 joules is frequently enough for cardioversion of ventricular tachycardia and 100 joules is almost always effective. If reversion fails, use stepwise increases of 25, 50, 100, 200, 300, and 400 joules. Myocardial injury and arrhythmias following cardioversion are directly related to the amount of energy delivered in a single shock and not to repeated shocks.

IV lines should be secured, and lidocaine given by slow infusion and bolus.

Variations

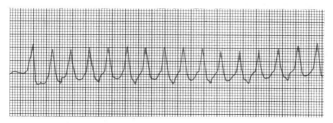

Ventricular tachycardia with retrograde conduction to the atria

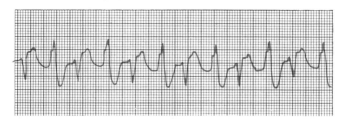

Bidirectional ventricular tachycardia

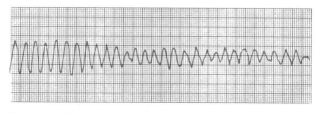

Ventricular flutter

Torsades de pointes (discussed on p. 72)

Differential Diagnosis

	Ventricular Tachycardia	Supraventricular Tachycardia with Aberrancy
AV dissociation	Present 50% of time	Absent
Axis	LAD	Inferior
QRS duration	>0.14 sec	0.14 sec or less
Morphology	If mainly upright in V_1: V_1 monophasic or biphasic V_6 S>R	V_1 triphasic (rSR')
	If mainly negative in V_1: V_1-V_2 R > 30 msec V_1-V_2 > 60 msec to nadir of S; notch in downstroke of S V_6 any Q	V_1-V_2 narrow R Sharp smooth downstroke of S V_6 monophasic R

Treatment

If there is hemodynamic deterioration, cardioversion is indicated; otherwise lidocaine or procainamide may be given. Begin cardioversion attempts with 10 watt-seconds and increase increments until successful.

Ventricular Fibrillation

Ventricular fibrillation is disorganized electrical activity in the ventricles, rendering them incapable of pumping blood.

Pathophysiology and Mechanism

Individual muscle fibers in the ventricles are depolarizing, but they are disorganized and fail to produce a proper ventricular contraction. The heart quivers and twitches, but does not pump (Fig. 4-2).

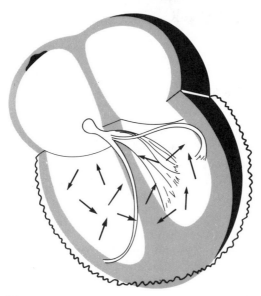

Figure 4-2
Ventricular fibrillation results when there is electrical chaos in the ventricles. It is initiated by a single PVC or is a deterioration of ventricular tachycardia.

ECG Characteristics

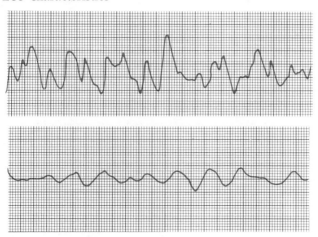

Rate: Not applicable
Rhythm: Not applicable
PR interval: Not applicable
QRS complex: Not applicable
Distinguishing features: An erratic fibrillatory line without QRS complexes

Causes

- Myocardial infarction
- Myocardial ischemia
- R-on-T, frequent, paired, or multifocal PVCs in the setting of acute myocardial infarction

Nursing Implications

The arrhythmia is instantly identified because of the absence of well-formed QRS complexes and because the patient loses consciousness. Administer oxygen.

Prepare to defibrillate.

Variations

Coarse ventricular fibrillation
Fine ventricular fibrillation

Differential Diagnosis

None

Treatment

1. Cough CPR, if patient awake and able to cough.
2. Defibrillate with 200 joules; repeat once if necessary.
3. If successful, administer lidocaine, a bolus and an infusion per protocol.
4. If VF persists, initiate chest compression and positive pressure ventilation. Start IV line.
5. Epinephrine 1:10,000, 5 to 10 ml (0.5 to 1 mg) IV or intratracheal.
6. After 30 to 60 sec of ventilation and chest compression, defibrillate with 300 to 400 joules; may repeat once.
7. Bretylium 5 mg/kg IV bolus. (Some authorities would begin this sooner.)

8. Sodium bicarbonate 1 mEq/kg IV push, especially if metabolic acidosis is documented by arterial blood gases.

9. If VF persists, attempt improvement on ventilation and oxygenation, continuous CPR, obtain arterial blood gases, further sodium bicarbonate administration guided by arterial blood gas results, if available. If not, repeat one-half dose in 10 min.

10. Repeat epinephrine 0.5 to 1 mg IV push.

11. Repeat defibrillation 300 to 400 joules.

12. Consider other drugs—magnesium, nitroglycerine, or additional bretylium.

13. Consider methods of "new CPR."

 ## Torsades de Pointes

Torsades de pointes (twists of points) is a polymorphous ventricular tachycardia associated with a prolonged QT interval.

Pathophysiology and Mechanisms

Unknown

ECG Characteristics

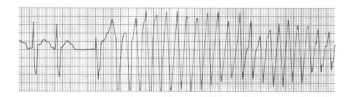

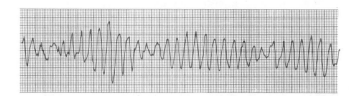

Rate: 150 to 250 beats/min
Rhythm: May be regular or irregular

PR interval: Not applicable

QRS complex: >0.12 sec and usually >0.14 sec

Distinguishing features: While in sinus rhythm the QT interval is too long (>0.46 to 0.50 sec or >33% of baseline). This measurement is absolute as opposed to corrected.

A ventricular tachycardia with phasic variation in the electrical polarity of the QRS complex.

The tachycardia may be paroxysmal, stopping, and then starting up again; the patient may be conscious.

Causes

Anything that lengthens the QT interval, such as the following:

- Antiarrhythmic drugs (quinidine, procainamide, disopyramide, or amiodarone)
- Hypokalemia
- Hypomagnesemia
- Profound bradycardia
- Intracerebral pathology
- Unilateral alteration of sympathetic tone
- Psychotropic drugs

Nursing Implications

Preventive care:

- Measure the QT interval on admission to the CCU.
- If the patient is on quinidine, procainamide, disopyramide, or amiodarone, alert all personnel to the importance of QT measurements.
- If possible, secure a QT measurement from a previous ECG.
- Notify the physician if the QT lengthens more than 33% or beyond 0.50 sec (not a corrected measurement).
- If torsades de pointes develops, prepare for pacing or IV magnesium sulfate.

Variations

None

Differential Diagnosis

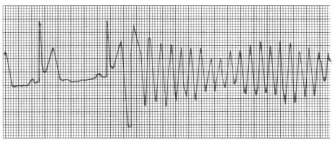

Coarse ventricular fibrillation without preceding QT lengthening; ventricular flutter

Treatment

Temporary overdrive ventricular or atrial pacing
IV magnesium sulfate (IV push: 2 g over 1 to 2 min; IV infusion: 1 to 2 g/hr for 4 to 6 hr)

Accelerated Idioventricular Rhythm

The accelerated idioventricular rhythm (AIVR) is an ectopic ventricular rhythm with a rate of 40 to 100 beats/min.

Pathophysiology and Mechanism

This arrhythmia is often seen in the setting of acute myocardial infarction and is thought to be benign unless it is the result of digitalis toxicity. The mechanism is enhanced automaticity.

ECG Characteristics

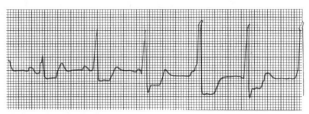

Rate: 40 to 100 beats/min
Rhythm: Regular

PR interval: Not applicable, but that of the underlying rhythm may be normal

QRS complex: >0.12 sec and usually >0.14 sec

Distinguishing features: A ventricular ectopic rhythm that often begins and ends with fusion beats and manifests itself when its rate is approximately that of the sinus node

Cause

▪ Acute myocardial infarction

Nursing Implications

This arrhythmia is identified and is not treated unless the accompanying AV dissociation is causing hemodynamic impairment.

Variations

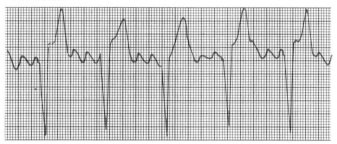

AIVR with atrial flutter

Treatment

Usually none

Ventricular Fusion Complexes

A ventricular fusion complex results when two impulses collide within the ventricles.

Pathophysiology and Mechanism

Ventricular fusion beats result from the presence of two opposing electrical currents (sinus and ventricular ectopic) within the same chamber at the same time. The resulting ECG complex is often narrower and of lesser amplitude than the ectopic beat alone. Ventricular fusion is often seen in association with ventricular parasystole, accelerated idioventricular rhythms, and end-diastolic PVCs.

ECG Characteristics

F

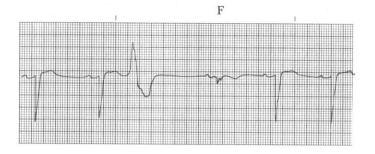

Rate: That of the underlying rhythm

Rhythm: Regular

PR interval: PR interval of the fusion beat may be the same as or shorter than that of the sinus rhythm, but is never more than 0.06 sec shorter than the dominant PR interval.

QRS complex: Normal in the underlying rhythm, but may be anything in the fusion beats

Distinguishing features: Other ventricular ectopic beats in the tracing and reason to believe that one was due at that moment.

QRS of the fusion beat has a contour intermediate between that of the fusing impulses.

Causes

▪ That of the ventricular ectopic beat or rhythm

Nursing Implications

In the setting of acute myocardial infarction, occasional ventricular fusion beats (end-diastolic PVCs) may warn of congestive heart failure. It is at this point in the cardiac cycle that the stretching of myocardial tissue is the greatest.

Generally, ventricular fusion beats have the nursing implications of the ventricular ectopic beat or rhythm itself.

Variations

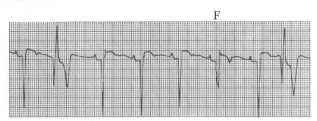

Ventricular parasystole

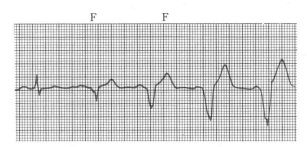

Accelerated idioventricular rhythm

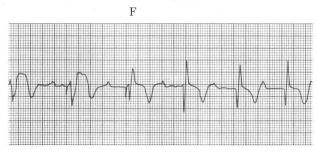

Electronic pacemaker fusion beat

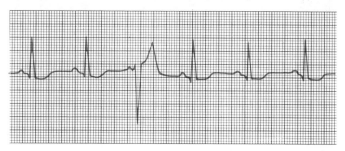

End-diastolic PVCs

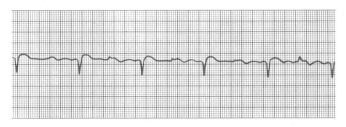

Bigeminal end-diastolic PVCs

Differential Diagnosis

Electrical alternans vs bigeminal end-diastolic PVCs

Treatment

Usually none

 Ventricular Parasystole

Ventricular parasystole is an independent and undisturbable ectopic rhythm whose pacemaker cannot be discharged by impulses of the dominant (usually sinus) rhythm.

Pathophysiology and Mechanism

Parasystolic rhythms develop because of an area of enhanced automaticity surrounded by an area of depressed tissue, which blocks any incoming impulses and keeps the pacemaker from being extraneously discharged. This protected ectopic pacemaker fires at regular intervals and captures the ventricles whenever they are nonrefractory; otherwise the beat goes undetected on the surface ECG (Fig. 4-3).

The parasystolic focus is not totally unresponsive to the electrical influence surrounding it and may be affected so that its rhythm is not precisely regular.

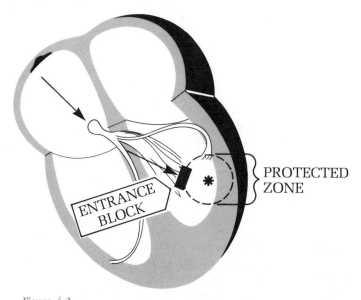

PROTECTED ZONE

ENTRANCE BLOCK

Figure 4-3
In ventricular parasystole there is a protected ectopic focus in the ventricles that keeps its own rate and is not discharged by extraneous impulses, although it may be electrogenically influenced by them.

ECG Characteristics

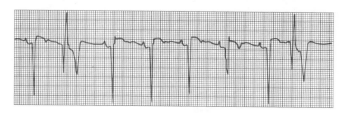

Rate: That of the underlying rhythm

Rhythm: Irregular, as a result of the extrasystoles

PR interval: Normal in the underlying rhythm

QRS complex: Normal in the underlying rhythm; broad in the parasystolic beats

Distinguishing features:

No fixed coupling

Interectopic intervals that have a common denominator

Fusion beats

Nursing Implications

The diagnosis is suspected when ventricular ectopics are observed without fixed coupling.

Since this is a benign arrhythmia, observe the patient for complications, but no treatment is indicated.

Even though it seems likely that a parasystolic beat will eventually activate the ventricles during the T wave, empirically when a parasystolic impulse coincides with the T wave it seldom becomes a manifest beat.

Variations

Fixed coupling in parasystole if the rates of the two pacemakers happen to be mathematically related

No fixed coupling, but interectopic intervals are not exact multiples, because the ectopic focus is influenced, but not reset, by the sinus impulses

Differential Diagnosis

Accelerated idioventricular rhythm

Treatment

Usually none

Ventricular Flutter

Ventricular flutter is a very rapid ventricular tachycardia without a clearly formed QRS complex.

Pathophysiology and Mechanism

This arrhythmia is a deterioration of ventricular tachycardia, representing severe disorganization within the ventricles.

ECG Characteristics

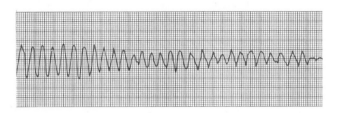

Rate: 150 to 300 beats/min
Rhythm: Regular or irregular
PR interval: Not applicable
QRS complex: Broad and poorly defined
Distinguishing features: A zig-zag, almost a sine wave configuration instead of clearly defined QRS complexes

Causes

- Myocardial infarction
- Myocardial ischemia
- R-on-T, frequent, paired, or multifocal PVCs in the setting of acute myocardial infarction
- An interim arrhythmia between ventricular tachycardia and fibrillation

Nursing Implications

This arrhythmia has the same clinical and nursing implications as ventricular tachycardia.

Variations

None

Differential Diagnosis

Torsades de pointes

Treatment

Same as for ventricular tachycardia

Ventricular Escape

Ventricular escape is characterized by an ectopic beat that originates in the ventricles and follows a long pause.

Pathophysiology and Mechanism

The ventricular escape beat is not abnormal in itself, but the fact that it is necessary is abnormal. Such a beat implies that (1) the sinus node or AV conduction failed, and (2) the junctional escape mechanism failed. A junctional escape beat is next in line after the sinus node for pacing function.

ECG Characteristics

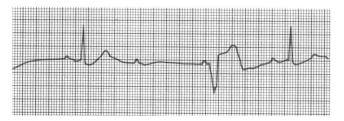

Rate: That of the underlying rhythm
Rhythm: Irregular
PR interval: Not applicable to this beat
QRS complex: Broad
Distinguishing features: A broad QRS that follows a long pause

Causes

- Failure of the sinus node or AV conduction along with failure of the junctional escape mechanism

Nursing Implications

The ventricular escape beat is a good thing in itself. Attention must be directed at (1) why there was not a normal sinus-conducted beat, and (2) why there was not a junctional escape beat instead of the ventricular escape.

Variations

None

Differential Diagnosis

Late junctional escape with phase 4 aberration

Treatment

That of the underlying problem

AV Block

5

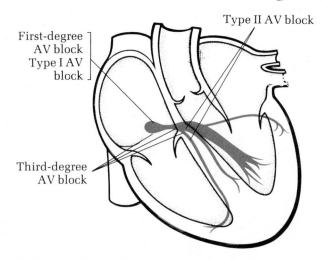

Type II AV block

First-degree
AV block
Type I AV
block

Third-degree
AV block

AV block is divided into first, second, and third degree. In first-degree AV block, all sinus impulses are conducted with delay. Second-degree AV block is either type I or type II. The only thing the two types have in common is dropped beats; the pathophysiology, clinical implications, treatment, and prognosis are completely different for the two. In third-degree AV block, no impulses reach the ventricles because of the presence of a pathological barrier.

Anatomy and Physiology

AV block is commonly located in the AV node, bundle of His, or bundle branches. Third-degree (complete) AV block may be located at any of the three levels. If the block is located in all three fascicles of the bundle branches, it is called "trifascicular block" (p. 112). In complete heart block, no impulses pass from atria to ventricle even when there is the opportunity to do so.

In type I AV block (Wenckebach), the pathology is at the level of the AV node, whereas in type II AV block the bundle branches are involved. In first-degree AV block the conduction delay may be anywhere from the atria to the bundle branches, but is usually in the AV node.

First-Degree AV Block

First-degree AV block is a consistent delay in AV conduction with all P waves being conducted and all PR intervals the same.

Pathophysiology and Mechanism

There is a delay in AV conduction usually at the level of the AV node, although the pathology could be anywhere from the atrium to the branching of the bundle of His.

ECG Characteristics

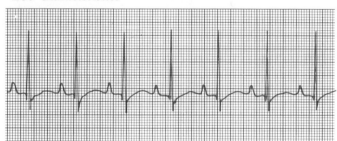

Rate: Normal
Rhythm: Regular
PR interval: >0.20 sec
QRS complex: Normal
Distinguishing features: Long PR with all beats conducted and an adequate R-P interval

Causes

- Digitalis
- Ischemic heart disease

- Inferior-wall myocardial infarction
- Hyperkalemia
- Acute rheumatic fever
- A normal variant

Nursing Implications

If the AV block is in the setting of acute inferior-wall myocardial infarction, it is usually transient but may worsen to Wenckebach or third degree with an idiojunctional pacemaker.

If the AV block is in the setting of anterior-wall myocardial infarction, it is usually more serious and may be part of a trifascicular conduction problem.

Variations

None

Differential Diagnosis

None, although attention needs to be paid to whether there is pathology or the PR lengthening is secondary to a short RP

III

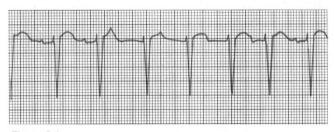

Figure 5-1
The reciprocal relationship between the RP interval and its complementing PR. The last four conducted beats demonstrate the converse of what happens in a Wenckebach: as the RP gets longer with each successive beat, its complementary PR gets progressively shorter, whereas in a Wenckebach the PR progressively lengthens in response to a progressively shortening RP.
(From Marriott, H.J.L., and Conover, M.H.B.: Advanced concepts in arrhythmias, St. Louis, 1983, The C.V. Mosby Co.)

interval. In Fig. 5-1 note that following the PAC, the PR lengthens for three cycles because of a short RP interval.

Treatment

None

Second-Degree AV Block

Type I (AV Nodal)

Type I AV block is incremental conduction delay at the level of the AV node until a P wave is not conducted (also called AV Wenckebach or Mobitz I).

Pathophysiology and Mechanism

AV nodal conduction is normally slow so that ischemia can easily cause incremental delay.

ECG Characteristics

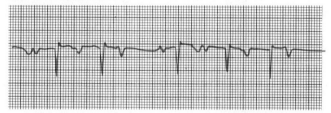

Rate: Normal
Rhythm: Irregular
PR interval: Lengthens until a beat is dropped. The first PR of the series is usually >0.20 sec.
QRS complex: Normal
Distinguishing features: Lengthening PR intervals, shortening RR intervals, and pauses that are less than twice the shortest cycle. There is group beating unless there is 2:1 conduction.

Causes

- Digitalis
- Ischemic heart disease

- Inferior-wall myocardial infarction
- Increased vagal tone, as in athletes

Nursing Implications

If the AV block is in the setting of acute inferior-wall myo-cardial infarction, it is usually transient but may worsen to third degree with an idiojunctional pacemaker.

Variations

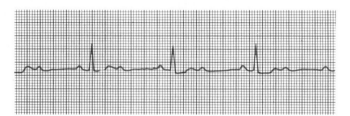

2:1 Wenckebach

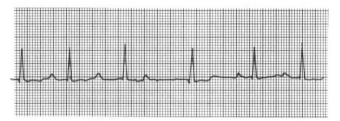

Wenckebach with junctional escape

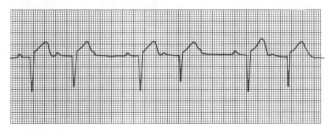

3:2 Wenckebach

Differential Diagnosis

Concealed junctional extrasystoles

2 : 1 AV conduction	Type I	Type II
PR	Long	Normal
QRS	Normal	Broad
Response to atropine	Yes	No

Treatment

None

Type II (Bundle-Branch)

Type II AV block is conduction delay at the level of the bundle branches.

Pathophysiology and Mechanism

There is a delay in AV conduction at the level of the bundle branches; therefore the QRS is usually broad. The PR is normal as long as conduction at the level of the AV node is not compromised as well.

ECG Characteristics

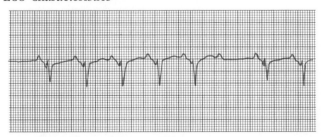

Rate: Normal
Rhythm: Irregular
PR interval: Normal, some P waves are not conducted
QRS complex: Broad
Distinguishing features: Fixed, normal PR intervals, broad QRS complexes, and dropped beats

Causes

- Severe conduction system disease
- Anterior-wall myocardial infarction

Nursing Implications

The diagnosis is made because there are nonconducted sinus P waves, the QRS is broad, and the PR intervals are normal.

This type of block is often irreversible and progresses into complete block.

The physician should be notified as Type II AV block may be an indication for a pacemaker.

Variations

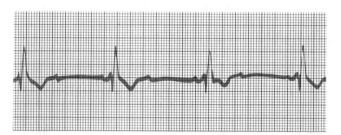

Type II with 2:1 AV conduction (other conduction ratios are possible)

Differential Diagnosis

Same as for type I

Treatment

Sometimes a pacemaker is indicated.

Third-Degree (Complete) AV Block

Third-degree, or complete, AV block is a pathological barrier to the passage of the atrial impulse into the ventricles.

Pathophysiology and Mechanism

There is pathology at the AV node, bundle of His, or bundle branches such that atrial impulses cannot pass. Thus the atria and the ventricles beat independently of each other.

ECG Characteristics

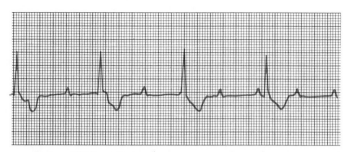

Rate: <58 beats/min

Rhythm: Regular

PR interval: Not applicable

QRS complex: Narrow or broad depending on the location of the escape pacemaker and the condition of the interventricular conduction system

Distinguishing features: Regular P waves at a rate of less than 130 beats min, regular QRS complexes at a rate of less than 58 beats/min, and AV dissociation

Causes

- Chronic degenerative conduction disease
- Digitalis toxicity
- Myocardial infarction

Nursing Implications

The diagnosis is made because of bradycardia, regular R waves, and regular P waves with AV dissociation

If the block is secondary to inferior-wall myocardial infarction, the escape pacemaker will be a dependable junctional one with a rate of about 55 to 58 beats/min. This is usually a reversible condition and a pacemaker may not be needed.

If the block is in the setting of acute anteroseptal myocardial infarction, the condition is usually more serious and irreversible.

In either case, the physician should be notified.

Variations

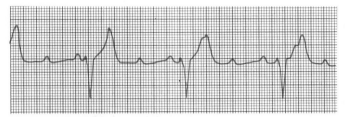

Third-degree AV block with an idioventricular rhythm (trifascicular block, see p. 112)

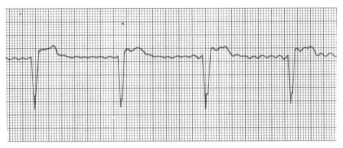

Atrial fibrillation with third-degree AV block

Differential Diagnosis

None

Treatment

A pacemaker is usually indicated in the setting of acute anterior-wall myocardial infarction.

AV Dissociation

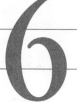

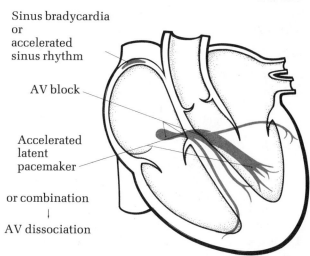

Sinus bradycardia
or
accelerated
sinus rhythm

AV block

Accelerated
latent
pacemaker

or combination
↓
AV dissociation

AV dissociation is the independent beating of atria and ventricles. It is important to remember that the term ''AV Dissociation'' is a hemodynamic consideration and not the ECG diagnosis. The primary disorder is indicated by the ECG diagnosis, which may be clinically insignificant, such as sinus bradycardia and junctional escape in an athlete, or it may be clinically significant, such as an accelerated idiojunctional rhythm or complete AV block. Thus the cause must always be identified.

Pathophysiology and Mechanism

AV dissociation is never a primary disorder, but always the result of a basic disturbance in impulse formation and/or conduction.

ECG Characteristics

Rate: That of the ventricular pacemaker

Rhythm: Usually regular but may be irregular if there is occasional conduction

PR interval: Not applicable

QRS duration: Narrow or broad, depending on the ventricular pacemaker

Distinguishing features: Independently beating atria and ventricles. In some cases the P waves may appear to "walk into" R waves.

Causes

- Sinus bradycardia
- Enhanced automaticity of a subsidiary pacemaker
- AV block
- Any combination of the above

Nursing Implications

The diagnosis is made because the ventricular rhythm is regular and independent of the P waves. Occasional shortening of the cycle length indicates capture (AV conduction).

Since the causes vary from normal conditions to abnormal ones, it is important to determine the mechanism and cause.

If the QRS complexes are narrow, the ventricular pacemaker is junctional (bundle of His). Determine the rate to find out if this represents a normal escape mechanism or an accelerated focus.

If the QRS complexes are broad, the ventricular pacemaker is ventricular or may be junctional with bundle-branch block.

If this is a normal escape mechanism, the only concern is hemodynamics.

If there is an accelerated idiojunctional focus, digitalis may be the cause, and the physician should be notified. Electrolyte and digitalis levels may be ordered.

An accelerated idioventricular focus is considered benign, and the patient only needs watching.

Variations

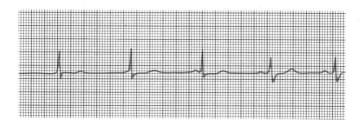

Sinus bradycardia with a junctional escape rhythm

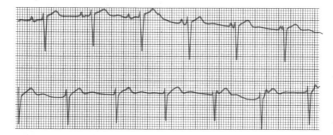

Accelerated idiojunctinal rhythm

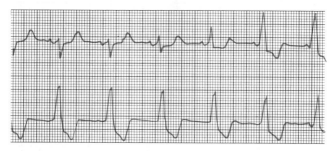

Accelerated idioventricular rhythm

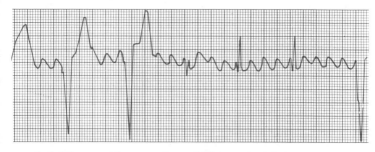

Atrial flutter with an accelerated idioventricular rhythm

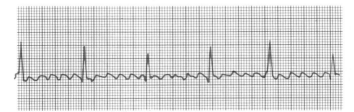

Atrial flutter with AV dissociation and 2 capture beats (first and fifth)

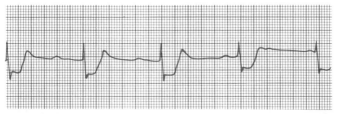

Complete AV block

C

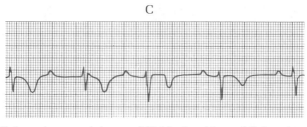

High-grade second-degree AV block with an idiojunctional pacemaker and one capture beat

Differential Diagnosis

See "Variations."

Treatment

If the AV dissociation is a result of an accelerated subsidiary pacemaker, a clinical assessment is indicated, and the cause is treated.

If there is sinus bradycardia with a junctional escape focus, no treatment may be indicated as long as there is no hemodynamic deterioration.

Bundle-Branch Block and Hemiblock

7

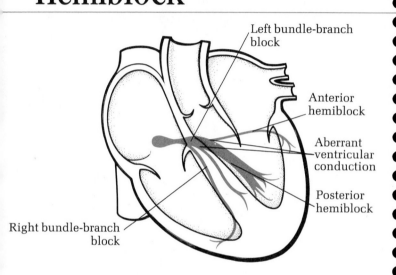

Left bundle-branch block

Anterior hemiblock

Aberrant ventricular conduction

Posterior hemiblock

Right bundle-branch block

A block at the level of the bundle branches results in right or left bundle-branch block (RBBB or LBBB), which causes the ventricles to be activated in sequence instead of simultaneously. This produces a long QRS complex that has a typical diagnostic morphology in V_1 and V_6. The left bundle branch is divided into two or three fascicles; a block of the main ones produces hemiblock.

Anatomy and Physiology

In normal intraventricular activation, both ventricles are activated at the same time, producing a narrow QRS. The bundle branches speed the impulse to the ventricles. Therefore when a bundle branch is blocked, the ventricle served by that bundle branch is activated late and the QRS is 0.12 sec or more. Hemiblock is a block of one division (anterior or posterior) of the left bundle branch.

Right Bundle-Branch Block
Pathophysiology and Mechanism

The right bundle branch is much smaller than the left and can be compromised by a lesser lesion. Thus RBBB is frequently clinically benign. When the right bundle branch is blocked, septal and left-ventricular activation are normal, but the impulse arrives under V_1 later than it should, causing the R wave to be later (late intrinsicoid deflection) in that lead (Fig. 7-1).

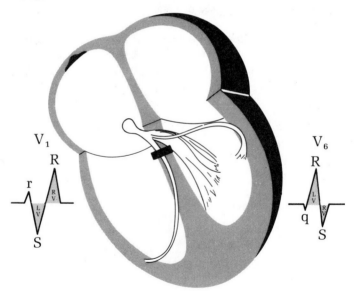

Figure 7-1
In RBBB, activation of both ventricles in sequence causes a broad complex with a late R wave in V_1 and an S wave in V_6.

ECG Characteristics

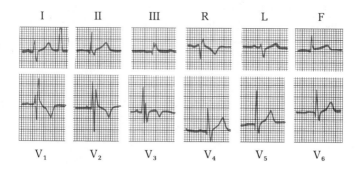

Rate: Normal
Rhythm: Normal
PR interval: Normal

QRS complex: 0.12 sec or greater; classical pattern in V_1 is rSR′

Distinguishing features: A broad QRS that is mainly positive in V_1 and has an intrinsicoid deflection of 0.07 sec or later in that lead. In I, aV_L, and V_6, the only abnormality is a broad S wave. There are secondary T wave changes.

Causes:

- Found in otherwise normal hearts
- Lenegre's disease
- Lev's disease
- Ischemic heart disease
- Chagas' disease
- Rheumatic disease
- Syphilis
- Trauma
- Tumors
- Cardiomyopathy
- Congenital lesions
- Surgical correction of tetralogy of Fallot or ventricular septal defect
- Acute heart failure
- Acute myocardial infarction

- Acute coronary insufficiency
- Acute infection
- Right-heart catheterization
- Intracardiac catheter in position

Nursing Implications

The diagnosis is made in V_1 because of a broad QRS that is mainly positive and has a late R wave.

In the setting of acute anteroseptal myocardial infarction, such a diagnosis is associated with a mortality of 65% and often the anterior division of the left bundle is also compromised. When bundle-branch block develops in this clinical setting the physician should be notified.

If the RBBB is in the setting of apparent health there is no adverse effect.

Variations

V_1

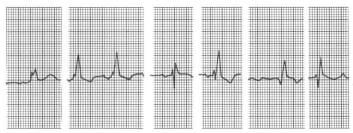

Different shapes of RBBB in V_1

V_1

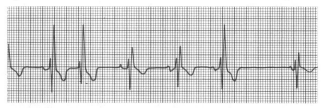

Incomplete RBBB has the QRS shape but not the duration.

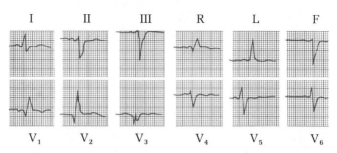

RBBB and anteroseptal myocardial infarction; anterior hemiblock is also present

V₁

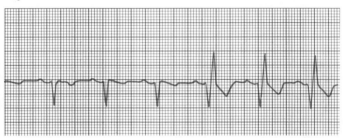

When the rate increases from 80 to 82 beats/min (the ''critical
rate''), rate-related RBBB results.

Differential Diagnosis

None

Treatment

None, although in the setting of acute anteroseptal myocardial
infarction, a pacemaker may be indicated

Left Bundle-Branch Block
Pathophysiology and Mechanism

LBBB (Fig. 7-2) usually reflects serious underlying heart disease because a large lesion is required to block the left bundle

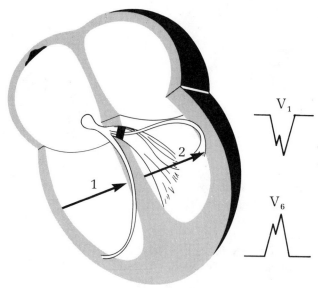

Figure 7-2

In LBBB, activation of both ventricles in sequence causes a very broad complex that is negative in V_1 and positive in V_6.

branch. This bundle is thick and broad and has a blood supply from two sources, the right and left coronary arteries. Typically the lesion is in the common left bundle before it branches.

When the left bundle branch is blocked, both initial and terminal forces are abnormal. The septum is activated from right to left; the left ventricle is activated from the currents in the right ventricle.

ECG Characteristics

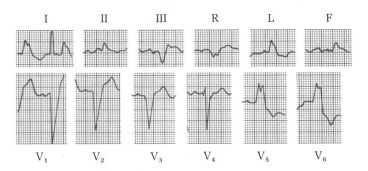

| I | II | III | R | L | F |

| V₁ | V₂ | V₃ | V₄ | V₅ | V₆ |

Rate: Normal
Rhythm: Normal
PR interval: Normal
QRS complex: 0.12 sec or greater
Distinguishing features: A broad QRS that is mainly negative in V_1. In I, aV_L, and V_6 there is an R wave, no q wave, and no S wave. There are secondary T wave changes.

Causes

- Found in otherwise normal hearts
- Lenegre's disease
- Lev's disease
- Ischemic heart disease
- Rheumatic disease
- Syphilis
- Trauma
- Tumors
- Cardiomyopathy
- Congenital lesions
- Severe aortic stenosis
- Acute heart failure
- Acute myocardial infarction
- Acute coronary insufficiency
- Acute infection

Nursing Implications

The diagnosis is made in V_1 because of a broad QRS that is mainly negative and in V_6 because of a broad R wave.

The physician should be notified if LBBB develops in the setting of acute anteroseptal myocardial infarction.

The prognosis depends on the underlying cause.

Variations

V_1

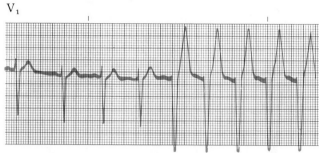

When the rate increases to 100 beats/min (the "critical rate"), rate-related LBBB results.

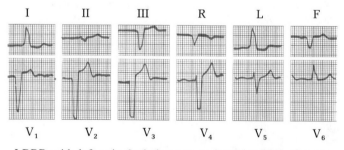

LBBB with left axis deviation occurs in about 30% of cases of LBBB. It is thought to indicate more extensive damage to the anterior fascicle of the left bundle.

Differential Diagnosis

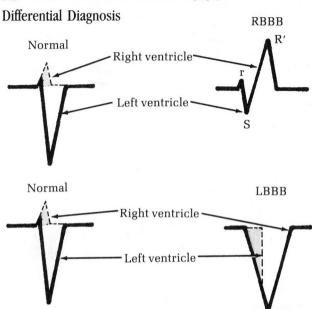

Normal conduction, right bundle-branch block, and left bundle-branch block compared in lead V_1. The dotted lines indicate hidden events on the ECG. For example, right-ventricular activation is normally effaced by left-ventricular activation.

Treatment

None, although in the setting of acute anteroseptal myocardial infarction, a pacemaker may be indicated

Anterior Hemiblock

Anterior hemiblock is a block of the anterior superior division of the left bundle branch.

Pathophysiology and Mechanism

Anterior hemiblock (Fig. 7-3) is more common and less serious than posterior hemiblock. The anterior fascicle of the

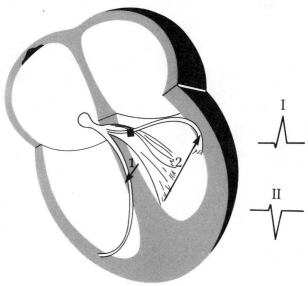

Figure 7-3
Left anterior hemiblock (LAH) causes left axis deviation.

LBB is long and thin, has only one blood supply, as does the RBB, and is in the outflow tract of the left ventrlcle, whereas the posterior fascicle is broad, has two blood supplies, and is not subjected to the mechanical stresses of the anterior division.

When the anterior fascicle is blocked, the impulse activates the ventricles via the posterior inferior fascicle; this produces left axis deviation.

ECG Characteristics

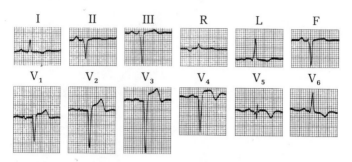

Rate: Normal
Rhythm: Normal
PR interval: Normal
QRS complex: Normal (lengthens by only 0.02 sec)
Distinguishing features:

Left axis deviation of more than -45 degrees (generally accepted)

A terminal R wave in aV_R and aV_L

The R wave in aV_R is later than the R in aV_L

A q wave in I and aV_L and an r wave in II, III, and aV_F

Increased QRS voltage in the limb leads

Causes

- Found in otherwise normal hearts
- Lenegre's disease
- Lev's disease
- Aortic valve calcification
- Cardiomyopathy
- Ischemic heart disease
- Acute myocardial infarction
- Cardiac catheterization
- Selective coronary arteriography
- Hyperkalemia
- Surgical correction of tetralogy of Fallot

Nursing Implications

The diagnosis is made because lead I is positive and lead II is negative, reflecting a left axis deviation of more than -45 degrees.

The physician should be notified if anterior hemiblock develops in the setting of acute anteroseptal myocardial infarction.

The prognosis depends on the underlying cause.

Variations

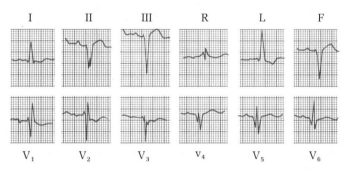

RBBB and anterior hemiblock

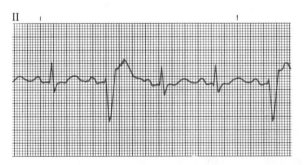

Intermittent anterior hemiblock with first-degree AV block and RBBB

Treatment

Usually none, although in the setting of acute anteroseptal myocardial infarction, a pacemaker may be indicated

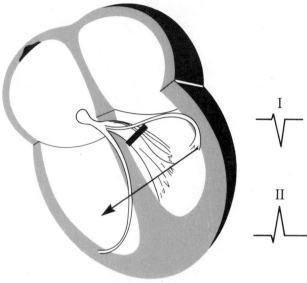

Figure 7-4
Left posterior hemiblock (LPH) has right axis deviation and is less common than LAH because the posterior fascicle has two blood supplies and the anterior only one.

 ## Posterior Hemiblock

Posterior hemiblock is a block of the posterior inferior division of the left bundle branch.

Pathophysiology and Mechanism

Posterior hemiblock (Fig. 7-4) has more serious clinical implications, because it implies the compromise of two blood supplies (right and left coronary arteris) and damage to a broad inferior conduction system in the left ventricle.

When the posterior fascicle is blocked, the impulse gets into the ventricles via the anterior superior fascicle; this produces right axis deviation.

ECG Characteristics

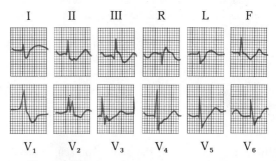

I   II   III   R   L   F

V_1 V_2 V_3 V_4 V_5 V_6

Rate: Normal, but may be accelerated or slow as a result of another conduction

Rythm: Normal

PR interval: Normal

QRS complex: Normal (lengthens by only 0.02 sec)

Distinguishing features:

Right axis deviation of more than +120 degrees

A q wave in II, III, and aV_F

An r wave in I and aV_L

Increased QRS voltage in the limb leads

Causes

- Lenegre's disease
- Lev's disease
- Aortic valve calcification
- Cardiomyopathy
- Ischemic heart disease
- Acute myocardial infarction
- Cardiac catheterization
- Selective coronary arteriography
- Hyperkalemia

Nursing Implications

The diagnosis is made because lead I is negative and lead II is positive, reflecting a right axis deviation of more than +120 degrees; be sure to rule out right-ventricular hypertrophy.

The physician should be notified if posterior hemiblock develops in the setting of acute anteroseptal myocardial infarction.

The prognosis depends on the underlying cause.

Variations

Usually, posterior hemiblock is accompanied by RBBB, which may be intermittent.

Treatment

Usually none, although in the setting of acute anteroseptal myocardial infarction, a pacemaker may be indicated

---

Trifascicular Block

Trifascicular block is a complete or incomplete pathological conduction impairment located simultaneously in the three main fascicles of the intraventricular conductive system—the right bundle branch and the anterior and posterior divisions of the left bundle branch (Fig. 7-5).

Pathophysiology and Mechanism

Pathology in three of the fascicles of the intraventricular conduction system is very ominous and implies compromise of two coronary arteries, the anterior descending left and the posterior descending right. The anterior descending left coronary artery supplies the RBB, the anterior division of the LBB, and part of the posterior division of the LBB, the remainder of which is supplied by the posterior descending right coronary artery.

If the block is complete across all fascicles (there are actually four), the escape pacemaker will be below that level and will therefore be a slow ventricular pacemaker whose rate is incompatible with life. If the block is not complete, then the supraventricular impulses arrive in the ventricles either with first-degree AV block type II second-degree AV block.

ECG Characteristics

Rate: That of the underlying rhythm; if complete block ventricular rate is < 40/min

Rhythm: That of the underlying rhythm

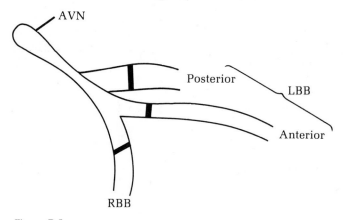

Figure 7-5

Trifascicular block. When this type of block is complete in all fascicles, complete AV block results.

PR interval: That of the underlying rhythm

QRS complex: Broad

Distinguishing features: This condition may take many forms:

Complete AV block

RBBB + LAH + first-or second-degree AV block

RBBB + LPH + first-or second-degree AV block

LBBB + first-or second-degree AV block

Various combinations of these

Causes

- Coronary artery disease
- Lenegre's disease
- Lev's disease

Nursing Implications

If the trifascicular block is complete, the patient suddenly plunges into profound bradycardia and emergency pacemaker insertion is indicated.

If the trifasicular block is incomplete (see ''Distinguishing Features,'' notify the physician and prepare for elective pacemaker insertion.

Variations

Complete AV block with a slow idioventricular rhythm
RBBB + LAH + first-degree or type type II second-degree
  AV block
RBBB + LPH + first-degree or type II second-degree AV
  block
LBBB + first-degree or type II second-degree AV block
Various combinations of these

Treatment

A pacemaker may be inserted.

Aberrancy vs Ectopy

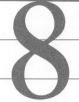

8

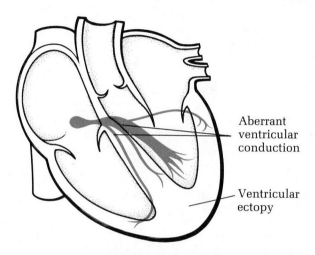

Aberrant ventricular conduction

Ventricular ectopy

Aberrant ventricular conduction is a transient bundle-branch block and/or hemiblock that is commonly though not exclusively caused by an abrupt shortening of cycle length. It is important to differentiate between aberrancy and ectopy, because the patient should not be given unnecessary medications nor should those he does need be withheld.

The differential diagnosis is based on the presence or absence of PACs preceding the broad beat, the shape of the QRS in V_1 and V_6, and the axis, the rate, the QRS duration, and the presence or absence of AV dissociation.

Pathophysiology and Mechanism

In aberrant ventricular conduction (Fig. 8-1), one or more of the main bundle branches or the fascicles may be blocked. Commonly this transient block occurs in the right bundle

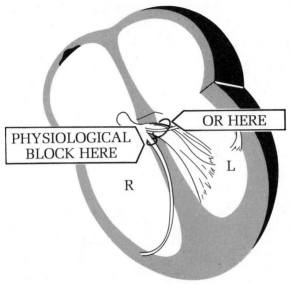

Figure 8-1
Aberrancy is the temporary abnormal conduction of a supraventricular complex.

branch but may also take the form of RBBB plus anterior or posterior hemiblock, hemiblock alone, or LBBB.

Ventricular ectopy commonly results from enhanced automaticity in the His-Purkinje system or from a microreentry circuit.

Nursing Implications

It is important that aberrancy be distinguished from ventricular ectopy so that the primary condition can be identified and treated. This is especially important in wide QRS tachycardia.

Morphology of the QRS

RBBB aberration (Fig. 8-2): Note the triphasic patterns in V_1 and V_6.

Ventricular ectopy (Figs. 8-3 and 8-4): Note the monophasic R or biphasic complex in V_1-V_2 and the QS or S larger than the R in V_6.

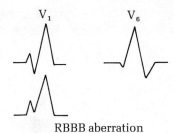

RBBB aberration

Figure 8-2

RBBB aberration. When these patterns are seen, RBBB aberration is indicated as long as the axis is not left.

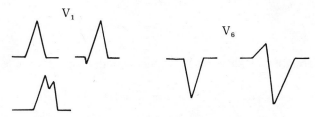

Figure 8-3

When the complex is mainly positive in V_1, ventricular ectopy is suggested when in V_1 there is a monophasic or biphasic complex, or "rabbit ears," or when in V_6 the S is bigger than the R.

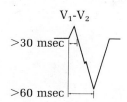

Figure 8-4

These signs are highly predictive of VT when the complex is mainly negative in V_1. Look for a broad R, notched S, and/or >60 msec to the nadir of the S wave.

Differential Diagnosis Between Supraventricular Tachycardia with Aberration and Ventricular Tachycardia

	Supraventricular Tachycardia	Ventricular Tachycardia
Axis	Normal	Left > − 30 degrees (unless there is left axis in sinus rhythm)
AV dissociation	No	Yes
Fusion beats	No	Occasional
Concordant QRS complex in the precordial leads	No	Occasional

Variations of Aberrant Ventricular Conduction

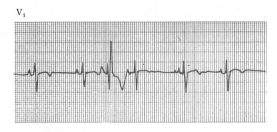

PAC with RBBB aberrancy

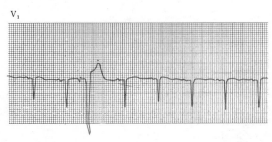

PAC with LBBB aberrancy

V₁

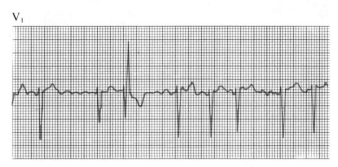

Atrial fibrillation with RBBB aberrancy

V₂

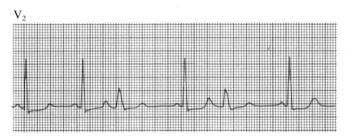

Bigeminal PACS with aberrancy

V₁

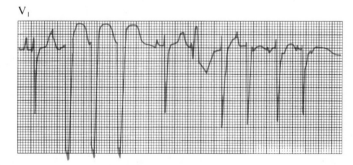

RBBB and LBBB aberrancy

V₁

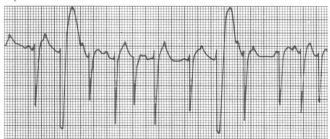

Chaotic atrial tachycardia with LBBB aberrancy

Variations of Ventricular Ectopy

V₁

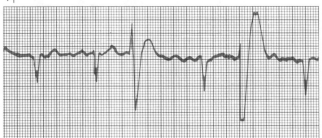

Atrial fibrillation with ventricular ectopics (Note the fat R wave.)

V₂

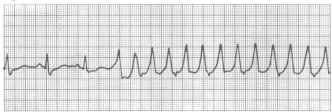

Ventricular tachycardia with 2:1 retrograde conduction to the atrium

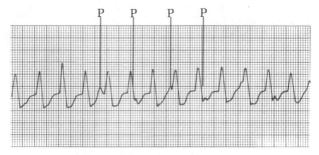

Ventricular tachycardia with AV dissociation (Regular, independent P waves during tachycardia are a sign of AV dissociation and support a diagnosis of ventricular tachycardia.)

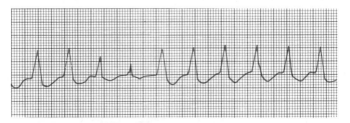

Ventricular tachycardia with ventricular fusion

Treatment

Aberrant ventricular conduction is not treated. The treatment
of ventricular ectopy is dictated by the clinical setting. In the
setting of acute myocardial infarction, lidocaine or procainamide is used.

Accessory Pathways

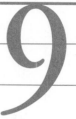

9

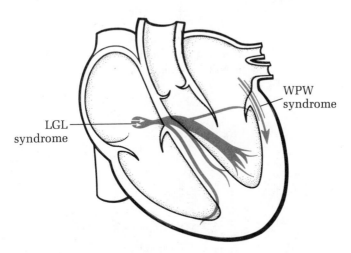

An accessory pathway is an extra muscle bundle between the atrium and the ventricle, which may cause a preexcitation syndrome. These patients are of interest because of their tendency to develop PSVT, which may deteriorate into atrial fibrillation or flutter with conduction down the accessory pathway and heart rates as high as 200 to 300 beats/min.

Classification of Accessory Pathways

There are three types of accessory pathways:

1. Accessory AV connection (Wolff-Parkinson-White syndrome): An extra muscle bundle forms a connection between atria and ventricles outside the conduction system

2. AV nodal fast pathway (Lown-Ganong-Levine syndrome): An intranodal fast pathway that is excessively fast
3. Mahaim fibers: Nodoventricular or fasciculoventricular tracts

---

Wolff-Parkinson-White Syndrome

In its traditionally described form, Wolff-Parkinson-White (WPW) syndrome is preexcitation of the ventricles over an AV accessory pathway, producing a typical ECG picture. Now, three types of the ''syndrome'' are described: overt, nonevident (latent), and concealed.

Preexcitation is activation of part of the ventricles earlier than would be possible had the activating impulse traveled via the normal pathway across the AV node and bundle of His; only the typical form of WPW syndrome involves preexcitation.

Pathophysiology and Mechanism

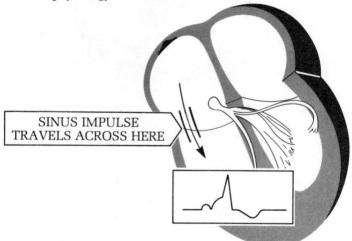

SINUS IMPULSE
TRAVELS ACROSS HERE

In *overt WPW syndrome,* there is preexcitation of the ventricles because of an accessory pathway connecting the atria and the ventricles, with conduction possible in both directions across it. This permits the sinus impulse to enter the ventricles without AV delay and outside of the conduction system, producing a short PR, a broad QRS, and a delta wave. This extra pathway may support a reentry circuit, as illustrated below, or provide rapid entry into the ventricles if atrial fibrillation or flutter should develop.

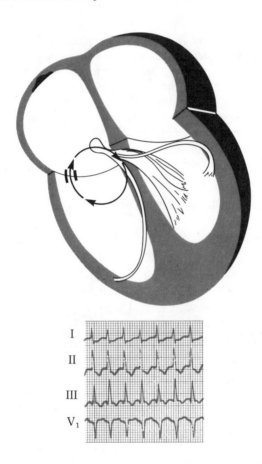

In *nonevident WPW syndrome* the ECG is normal because the impulse crosses the AV node quicker than it crosses the accessory pathway.

In overt and nonevident WPW, there is a tendency to PSVT because the two separate AV pathways create a favorable environment for reentry. During atrial fibrillation conduction is over an accessory pathway as shown below; the resultant rhythm is fast, broad, and irregular (FBI). Although patients with *concealed WPW syndrome* suffer from PSVT, it has recently been found by Wellens' group that they do not develop atrial fibrillation. The reason for this is not known.

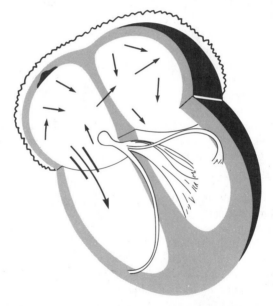

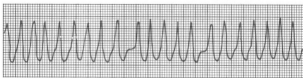

ECG Characteristics

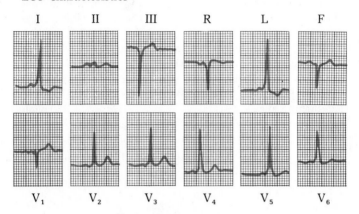

Overt WPW Syndrome
  Rate: Normal
  Rhythm: Regular
  PR interval: <0.12 sec
  QRS complex: >0.11 sec

Distinguishing features: Short PR, broad QRS, delta wave (slurred beginning to the QRS), and a tendency to PSVT and atrial fibrillation or flutter. There may be secondary T wave changes.

Nonevident WPW Syndrome
  Rate: Normal
  Rhythm: Regular
  PR interval: Normal
  QRS complex: Normal

Distinguishing features: Normal PR, normal QRS, and a tendency to PSVT and atrial fibrillation or flutter

Concealed WPW Syndrome
  Rate: Normal
  Rhythm: Regular
  PR interval: Normal
  QRS complex: Normal

Distinguishing features: Normal PR, normal QRS, and a tendency to PSVT

Cause

- Congenital

Nursing Implications

Unless there are arrhythmias associated with the presence of accessory pathways, there are no nursing implications.

Often the patient comes to the emergency room with PSVT or atrial fibrillation or flutter with conduction over the accessory pathway and very rapid ventricular rates, which may deteriorate into ventricular fibrillation.

If PSVT is the presenting symptom, the treatment is as listed on p. 128. However, once a sinus rhythm has been restored and the PR and QRS seem to be normal, the presence of an accessory pathway must be ruled out. The nurse must carefully examine the tracings taken during the tachycardia (see "Differential Diagnosis") to see if there are clues to the existence of an accessory pathway.

If atrial fibrillation with conduction over an accessory pathway is the presenting symptom, the rhythm will be so fast that emergency cardioversion is indicated. However, once the patient is stabilized the detective work begins. If there is a short PR, a broad QRS, and a delta wave while the heart is in sinus rhythm, the diagnosis is straightforward. If the PR and the QRS are normal, do not automatically assume that you have cardioverted a ventricular tachycardia. Atypical or concealed WPW syndrome is a definite possibility. Examine the tracings of the tachycardia carefully. If there was atrial fibrillation with conduction over an accessory pathway, the rate will be 200 to 300 beats/min, the QRS complexes will be broad, and the rhythm will be irregular.

Variations

Overt WPW
Nonevident WPW
Concealed WPW

Differential Diagnosis

The tachycardia secondary to atrial fibrillation with conduction over an accessory pathway must be differentiated from ventricular tachycardia, since both have broad QRS complexes.

	Ventricular Tachycardia	Atrial Fibrillation in WPW Syndrome
Rate	<170 beats/min	>200 beats/min
Rhythm	Regular	Irregular
QRS complex	Broad	Broad

Remember the easy clue to the diagnosis of atrial fibrillation in WPW syndrome: FBI (fast, broad, irregular).

If atrial flutter develops there is a 1:1 response and activation is across the accessory pathway, so the QRS is broad.

ECG Differential Diagnosis Between CMT and AVN Reentry

ECG Sign	CMT	AVN Reentry
P' waves	Between the R waves	Hidden in QRS or peeking out at end
Initiating P'R	Not abnormally long	Long
QRS alternans	Present 30% of time	Very rare after first 5 seconds
Aberrancy	Common	Rare

Always secure five leads (I, II, III, V_1, V_2) while the patient is in the PSVT, as P waves may be seen in one lead and not in another. In CMT the P' wave is separate from the QRS and usually closest to the preceding R (comparison with the sinus rhythm helps).

During aberrant ventricular conduction, the heart rate is slower than without aberrancy if the accessory pathway is on the same side as the bundle branch block aberration.

Treatment

PSVT:

Use a vagal maneuver.

If unsuccessful, cardioversion, verapamil, or procainamide is indicated, depending on the hemodynamic status of the patient and the clinical judgment of the physician.

Atrial fibrillation and a rapid, irregular ventricular rate:

Cardioversion

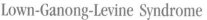

Lown-Ganong-Levine Syndrome

Lown-Ganong-Levine (LGL) syndrome is preexcitation of the ventricles over a fast AV internodal pathway; it produces a typical ECG picture.

Pathophysiology and Mechanism

There is a pathway within the AV node that conducts the impulse very rapidly, producing the typical ECG and leaving the patient vulnerable to PSVT resulting from AV nodal reentry. The shorter the PR the more likely it is that the fast pathway will be capable of sustaining AV nodal reentry.

ECG Characteristics

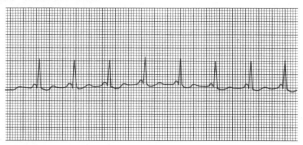

Rate: Normal
Rhythm: Regular
PR interval: <0.12 sec
QRS complex Normal
Distinguishing features: Short PR, normal QRS, and a tendency to PSVT and atrial fibrillation or flutter

Nursing Implications

This condition is usually easily diagnosed. If the patient has a tendency to PSVT, atrial fibrillation, and atrial flutter, the hemodynamic compromise during the arrhythmias may be very severe, and sudden death may result because of rapid ventricular rates.

Variations

None

Differential Diagnosis

None

Treatment of the PSVT

Same as for PSVT of WPW syndrome

Mahaim Fibers

Mahaim fibers are anomalous tracts between the AV node or bundle of His and the ventricles.

Pathophysiology and Mechanism

There are two main anatomic types of Mahaim fibers: nodo-ventricular and fasciculoventricular (Fig. 9-1). The nodoventricular fibers may or may not result in an abnormal ECG and are probably the tract that supports an AV reentry circuit.

ECG Characteristics

Rate: Normal
Rhythm: Regular
PR interval: May be short or normal
QRS complex: Varies in morphology
Distinguishing Features: A tendency to PSVT and atrial fibrillation or flutter. ECG picture depends on the origin and insertion of the extra fiber, as well as its length.

Causes

■ Congenital

Nursing Implications

Tendency to PSVT, atrial fibrillation, and atrial flutter
Hemodynamic compromise while the patient is in PSVT
Sudden death, because the PSVT has deteriorated into ventricular fibrillation

Variations

None

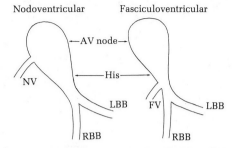

Site of origin: AV node · His bundle or bundle branches
PR: Short or normal · Normal (isolated FV)
QRS: Anomalous—fusion · Anomalous—fixed

Figure 9-1

Diagrammatic representation of the AV node and the two main varieties of Mahaim fibers. Nodoventricular *(NV)* fibers arise from the AV node itself, while fasciculoventricular *(FV)* fibers arise from the bundle of His or the bundle branches. (From Gallagher, J.J., and others: Role of Mahaim fibers in cardiac arrhythmias in man, Circulation **64**:176, 1981. By permission of the American Heart Association, Inc.)

Differential Diagnosis

WPW syndrome

Treatment of the PSVT

Same as for PSVT of WPW syndrome

Myocardial Infarction

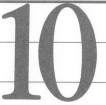

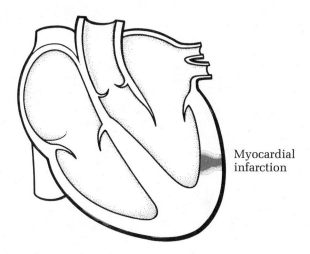

Myocardial
infarction

Myocardial infarction (MI) may be either transmural or sub-endocardial. The evolving MI will progress through ischemia and injury, which are reversible, to necrosis, which is not. The pathology is reflected as inverted T waves, elevated ST segments, and pathological Q waves in the ECG leads over the infarct. The leads on the wall opposite the infarct may exhibit reciprocal changes, that is, depressed ST segments, tall R waves, and tall T waves. (These may indicate more extensive pathology.)

Pathophysiology and Mechanism

Following a coronary occlusion cellular changes begin immediately because of ischemia. If the ischemic condition is severe and/or prolonged, the area of ischemic tissue becomes

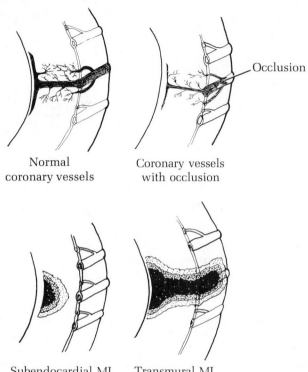

Normal
coronary vessels

Coronary vessels
with occlusion

Occlusion

Subendocardial MI   Transmural MI

Figure 10-1

more and more severely injured, cell functions cease, and irreversible cell injury ensues, producing a mass of necrotic
tissue. When this point is reached, the term ''myocardial infarction'' applies.

Injured tissue is unable to contract but may be able to re-
main in a viable and salvageable condition for some time and
may return to normal if collateral circulation develops and/or
blood flow improves in the area. However, if ischemia is very
severe and blood flow greatly impaired, cell death is inevita-
ble.

Myocardial infarction may involve the full thickness of the
ventricular wall, from endocardium to epicardium *(transmu-*

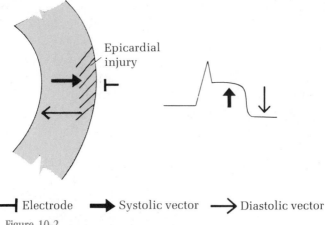

Epicardial injury

— Electrode   ➡ Systolic vector   → Diastolic vector

Figure 10-2
Effect of systolic and diastolic injury vectors on the ST segment because of epicardial injury.
(Modified from Surawicz, B., and Saito, S.: Am. J. Cardiol. **41:**943, 1978.)

ral), or only the inner layer of the ventricle *(subendocardial)* (Fig. 10-1).

Abnormal Q waves are seen in transmural MI in the leads directly over the infarcted tissue; they are the result of a loss of electrical potentials because of the severe injury. The more leads in which abnormal Q waves are seen, the larger the infarction. Q waves may persist indefinitely, or they may disappear months or years following an infarction.

ST segment elevation, along with the clinical picture and abnormal Q waves, is the sign of the acute evolving transmural infarction. Because of severe ischemia and lack of nutrients, the tissue immediately surrounding the center of the infarct is nonfunctional. It receives its blood supply from the collateral circulation. This is sufficient to keep it alive but insufficient to maintain membrane integrity, and because this tissue has a different membrane potential from the rest of the ventricle, a current of injury flows during repolarization (electrical systole) and/or during the resting phase (electrical diastole) to produce ST segment elevation (Fig. 10-2).

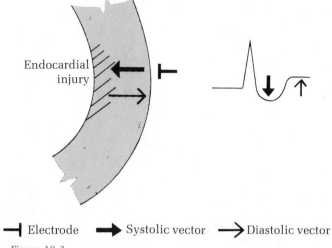

→| Electrode   ➡ Systolic vector   → Diastolic vector

Figure 10-3
Effect of systolic and diastolic injury vectors on the ST segment because of endocardial injury.
(Modified from Surawicz, B., and Saito, S.: Am. J. Cardiol., **41**:943, 1978.)

ST segment depression, along with the clinical picture, is the sign of subendocardial infarction. The systolic and diastolic currents of injury are in the opposite direction to what they are when the infarct involves the epicardium. Thus ST segment depression is produced (Fig. 10-3).

Deep T wave inversion occurs in leads reflecting ischemic tissue, because in such tissue the depolarization process is delayed and so is repolarization, causing T wave inversion (Fig. 10-4).

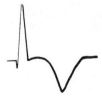

Figure 10-4
The typical coved ST and inverted T wave of evolving transmural infarction.

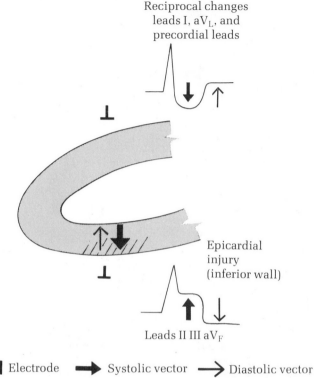

Reciprocal changes
leads I, aV$_L$, and
precordial leads

Epicardial
injury
(inferior wall)

Leads II III aV$_F$

⊣ Electrode   ➡ Systolic vector   → Diastolic vector

Figure 10-5
Reciprocal changes. Note the effect of systolic and diastolic
injury vectors on the ST segment in leads facing the wall
opposite the injury.

Fig. 10-5 illustrates reciprocal changes in inferior-wall MI,
in which case there are elevated ST segments in the inferior
leads (II, III, and aV$_F$) in the acute phase. If an ECG is ob-
tained early enough, it will often show ST depression in leads
facing the noninfarcted opposite wall (I, aV$_L$, and V$_1$ to V$_6$).
Just as the ST elevation seen in the inferior leads is the result
of an injury current flowing toward the reflecting leads, the
ST depression may be the result of this same current of injury

flowing away from the leads on the opposite side of the heart. Recent studies indicate that although such changes may be purely "reciprocal," more often they indicate a larger infarction involving the posterolateral or inferoseptal areas.

In true posterior-wall MI, there are no leads over the involved area; thus the ECG diagnosis depends on reciprocal changes in the leads over the opposite wall, V_1 to V_4. When posterior forces are lost, there is a gain in anterior forces. Thus instead of abnormal Q waves there will be tall R waves. The current of injury will produce depressed ST segments instead of elevated ones because it is being sensed from the opposite wall. Ischemia will be reflected by tall, pointed T waves instead of inverted ones. Recent studies comparing the surface ECG with motion studies of the heart indicate that the combination of a Q in II, III, aV_F, and V_6 and an R greater than S and a positive T wave in V_1 reflects inferoposterior infarct.

ECG Characteristics

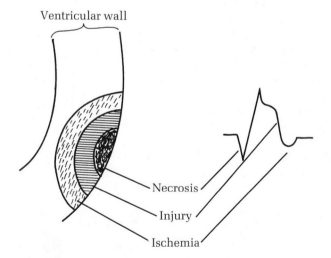

Ventricular wall

Necrosis

Injury

Ischemia

ECG signs of MI are supported by the clinical picture and an evolving picture as seen in serial tracings. The diagnosis is never made on the basis of the ECG alone.

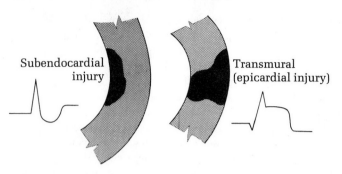

Subendocardial injury   Transmural (epicardial injury)

Transmural MI
- Abnormal Q waves: Present
- ST segments: Elevated
- T waves: Deeply inverted, typically coved

Subendocardial MI
- Abnormal Q waves: None
- ST segments: Depressed
- T waves: Inverted in several limb and precordial leads

True posterior-wall MI
- Abnormal Q waves: V_6; R $\geq$ S:V
- ST segments: May be depressed in V_1 to V_4 (a reciprocal change)
- T waves: May be tall and pointed in V_1 to V_4 (a reciprocal change)

Right-ventricular MI
- Abnormal Q waves: None, unless associated with inferior-wall MI
- ST segments: Elevation of 1 mm or more in right precordial leads V_{4R} to V_{6R} early in course of infarct
- T waves: Inverted in inferior leads if associated with inferior-wall MI

Nursing Implications

The diagnosis of acute MI is made because of the signs and symptoms and the elevated ST segments on the ECG. Note that as many as 25% of patients with acute MI have normal enzymes at the time they are seen in the emergency room.

In the emergency room, before transfer to the CCU:

1. Reassure the patient (anxiety can cause more PVCs).
2. Administer oxygen.
3. Establish an intravenous route.
4. Give prophylactic lidocaine (infusion and bolus) according to the hospital protocol.
5. Monitor the heart rhythm.
6. Relieve pain. If morphine is given, small increments will reduce the danger of hypotension, vagotonia, or respiratory depression. If hypotension develops, raise the feet. Vagotonia may require atropine, 0.3 to 1 mg. Respiratory depression may be reversed with naloxone (Narcan).

In the CCU, protect the patient from life-threatening arrhythmias. When there is ischemic and injured tissue in the heart, the ventricular fibrillatory threshold is lower and there are more ventricular ectopics.

Assess the hemodynamic status of the patient frequently. Because of the loss of contracting ventricular muscle, there will be a fall in cardiac output and the threat of congestive heart failure.

Secure the V_{4R} lead. Half of all patients with right-ventricular MI will develop AV conduction problems. Thus it is important to secure the V_{4R} tracing within the first 10 hours; frequently the elevated ST segment in this lead disappears after this time.

Variations

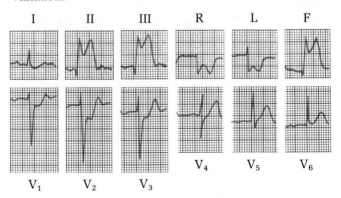

Inferior-wall MI

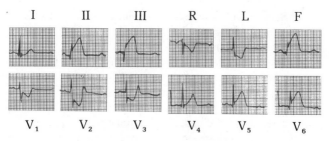

Inferoposterolateral MI

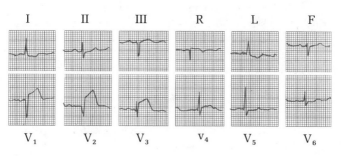

Anteroseptal MI

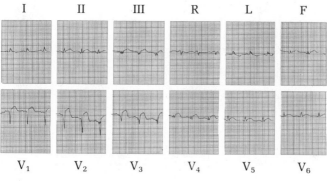

Anterior-wall MI (anterolateral)

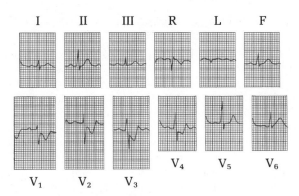

True posterior-wall MI

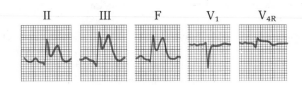

Inferior and right-ventricular wall MI

Differential Diagnosis

Type of Infarct	Indicative Changes (Q, ST elevation, T inversion)
Inferior	Q in II, III, aV_F
Inferoposterior	Q in II, III, aV_F, and V_6; R>S and positive T in V_1
Anteroseptal	V_1 to V_4
Antero to posterolateral	V_1 to V_5; Q in I, aV_L, and V_6
Posterior	V_1, R>S, positive T, and Q in V_6
Right ventricular	ST elevation in V_{4R}

Q waves resulting from causes other than MI

Normal variant. A QS complex may be normal in V_1 and in leads III and aV_F. In the electrically vertical heart, there may be a QS or Qr pattern in aV_L.

Infiltrative myocardial disease (such as amyloidosis), muscular dystrophy, and any other types of myocardial injury that cause a loss of electrical potentials and an inability to depolarize

Intraventricular conduction problems, such as in bundle-branch block and Wolff-Parkinson-White syndrome

Ventricular hypertrophy. In the leads facing the ventricle opposite to the hypertrophy, reciprocal Q waves may be seen.

ST-T changes not resulting from MI (partial list)

Prinzmetal's angina. An episode of chest pain associated with ST elevation that reverts to normal within a matter of minutes. The more common type is associated with diffuse depression of the ST segment with reciprocal ST elevation in aV_R.

Ventricular aneurysm. Causes persistent ST segment elevation after acute infarction because of a current of injury generated from the myocardial cells bordering the aneurysm.

Artifact, such as a wandering baseline.

T wave inversions resulting from causes other than ischemia

Normally inverted in aV_R

May be normally inverted or upright in V_1

Varies in V_2 and III

Normally positive in aV_L and aV_F, but may be inverted if the QRS is less than 6 mm tall

Normal variant in young black men, in athletes, and in the right-chest to midchest leads of children—the juvenile T wave pattern, which may persist to adulthood, especially in young black women

Secondary to bundle-branch block and Wolff-Parkinson-White syndrome, but their contour will be normal (asymmetrical and rounded)

Cerebrovascular accident: deeply inverted, wide, blunted T waves

Following bouts of tachycardia and artificial pacing

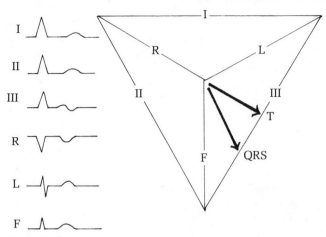

Figure 10-6

Method for plotting the T-wave axis. Lead III has zero net enclosed area, and therefore the mean T vector is perpendicular to the axis of lead III. Since aV_R has an axis perpendicular to III, it is this lead that will tell you the direction of the mean T vector. The T in aV_R is negative; thus the T axis is +30 degrees. Since the QRS axis is +60 degrees, the angle between the T and the QRS is 30 degrees.

Artifact produced either by the cardiac monitor (its filter) or by sloppy application of electrode paste across the chest

Method for plotting T wave axis

The angle between the axes of the QRS and the T wave is usually not over 45 degrees in the frontal plane or 60 degrees in the horizontal plane. The T axis is plotted in the same way as the QRS axis (Fig. 10-6).

Treatment (Initial Management)*

Morphine for the control of pain
Lidocaine to control ventricular ectopics
IV furosemide for fluid overload
Fluids for patients with right-ventricular infarction

*Adapted from Goldhaber, S.Z.,and Wold, M.A.: Chest pain. In May, H.L., editor: Emergency Medicine, New York, 1984, John Wiley & Sons.

Nitroprusside for marked hypertension (do not let blood pressure deviate more than 30 mm Hg from baseline)

Appropriately treat marked bradycardia, atrial fibrillation, or flutter and a rapid ventricular response

Transfer expeditiously from emergency room to CCU

Wellens' Syndrome

Wellens' syndrome is a group of six signs of critical stenosis of the proximal left anterior descending coronary artery. The signs are as follows:

- Prior angina
- Little or no enzyme elevation
- No Q wave
- Little or no ST elevation
- ST-T angle 60°-90°
- Deeply inverted symmetrical T wave

V_2-V_3

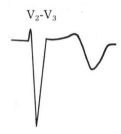

Warns of critical
LAD stenosis

Chamber Enlargement

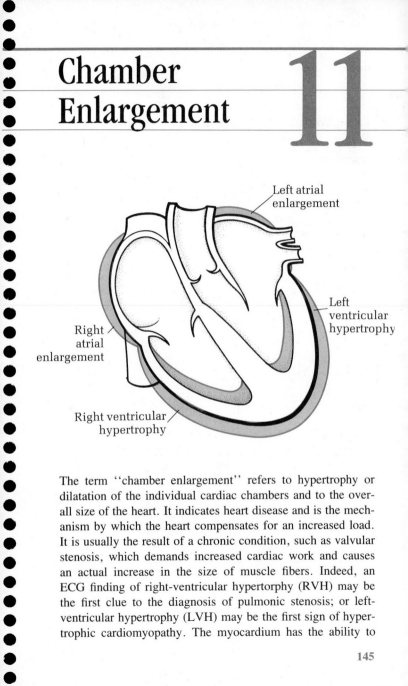

11

Left atrial enlargement

Left ventricular hypertrophy

Right atrial enlargement

Right ventricular hypertrophy

The term ''chamber enlargement'' refers to hypertrophy or dilatation of the individual cardiac chambers and to the overall size of the heart. It indicates heart disease and is the mechanism by which the heart compensates for an increased load. It is usually the result of a chronic condition, such as valvular stenosis, which demands increased cardiac work and causes an actual increase in the size of muscle fibers. Indeed, an ECG finding of right-ventricular hypertorphy (RVH) may be the first clue to the diagnosis of pulmonic stenosis; or left-ventricular hypertrophy (LVH) may be the first sign of hypertrophic cardiomyopathy. The myocardium has the ability to

145

increase its protein content by as much as 50% in response to such demands.

Left-Ventricular Hypertrophy
Pathophysiology and Mechanism

Increased QRS amplitude. When the left-ventricular wall hypertrophies, the disproportion in size between the left and right ventricles is increased, resulting in greater QRS amplitude, but a normal sequence of depolarization is retained (Fig. 11-1).

Intrinsicoid deflection. This component of the QRS complex (the peak of the R wave) reflects the time it takes for peak voltage to develop under that particular electrode. Because there is more muscle mass, this deflection is delayed in V_6 (Fig. 11-2).

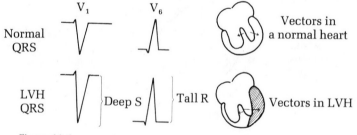

Figure 11-1
The normal QRS compared with that in LVH.

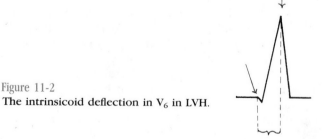

Figure 11-2
The intrinsicoid deflection in V_6 in LVH.

0.05 sec or more

Axis. The axis in LVH is normal because the conduction sequence is normal. As the heart hypertrophies, it rotates counterclockwise (posteriorly), producing a horizontal axis. A marked left axis shift suggests left anterior hemiblock, which may result from myocardial fibrosis secondary to longstanding hypertension.

"Strain" pattern. The mechanism is unknown but it correlates with increasing left-ventricular mass. It is known to be associated with longstanding LVH and to intensify when dilation and failure develop.

ECG Characteristics (see also Table 11-1)

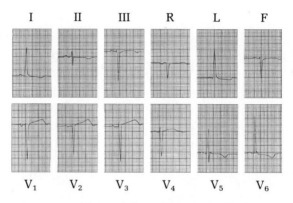

Note that the sensitivity of the ECG is limited in LVH.

Rate: Normal

Rhythm: Normal

PR interval: Normal

QRS complex: Increased amplitude. However, QRS voltage:

1. varies with age (greater in the young).
2. is normally greatest in the lead whose axis is parallel with the main current flow (electrical axis).
3. is greater in individuals with a thin chest wall.
4. is less in the obese individual and lung disease.

Distinguishing features:

Taller R waves in the left precordial leads

Deeper S waves in the right precordial leads

Table 11-1   Estes scoring system for left-ventricular hypertrophy*

1. Voltage criteria
Any of:
    a. R or S wave in limb leads = 20 mm
    b. S wave in V_1 or V_2 = 30 mm
    c. R wave in V_5 or V_6 = 30 mm
		3 points

2. ST-T abnormalities
    Without digitalis
    With digitalis
		3 points
		1 point

3. Left atrial abnormality
    Negative area under P wave in lead V_1
    ≥ 1 mm^2 (1 box)
		3 points

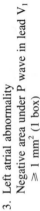

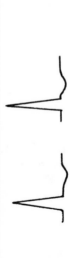

0.04 sec × −1.0 mm = −0.04 (abnormal)

4. Left axis deviation   2 points
5. QRS duration—.09 sec   1 point

6. Intrinsicoid deflection V_5 or $V_6 \geqslant .05$ sec   1 point

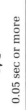

0.05 sec or more

*5 points, diagnostic; 4 points, probable.

Intrinsicoid deflection delayed in V_6 to 0.05 sec or more (measured from the onset of the QRS to the peak of the R wave)

Axis is normal

"Strain" pattern: ST-T-U abnormalities in V_5 and V_6. The ST segment is depressed with an upward convexity. The downward curve of the ST segment becomes an inverted T wave. U waves often invert.

Associated left-atrial enlargement

Causes

- Hypertension
- Aortic stenosis
- Aortic insufficiency
- Coarctation of the aorta
- Hypertrophic cardiomyopathy
- Athletics
- Myocardial infarction

Nursing Implications

The ECG signs of cardiac enlargement or hypertrophy are not sensitive, although they are specific.

The nursing care is supportive; the condition is a manifestation of another condition. There will be cardiac dysfunction because of increasing ventricular stiffness, elevated ventricular pressure, decreased passive ventricular filling, and decreased coronary blood flow, all of which will compound the seriousness should the patient sustain a myocardial infarction.

The patient may have a predisposition to subendocardial ischemia, and, if there is outflow tract obstruction, syncope frequently can occur because of an absent pressure gradient between the body of the left ventricle and the subaortic chamber.

Differential Diagnosis

See "Causes."

Treatment

That of the primary disease

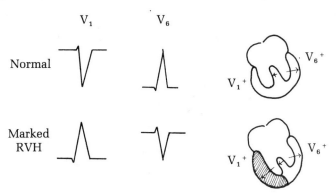

Figure 11-3
The normal QRS compared with that in RVH.

Right-Ventricular Hypertrophy
Pathophysiology and Mechanism

Normally the electrical forces of the thicker left ventricle dominate those of the right ventricle so that an rS appears in V_1 and a qR in V_5 and V_6. In *marked* right-ventricular hypertrophy the right ventricle dominates, there is right axis deviation, and the precordial pattern reverses (a tall R wave appears in V_1 and a deep S wave in V_6). A normal sequence of depolarization is retained (Fig. 11-3).

ECG Characteristics

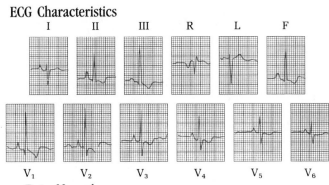

Rate: Normal
Rhythm: Normal

PR interval: Normal

QRS complex: Normal, but Q waves may develop in II, III, and aV_F

Distinguishing features:

Right axis deviation of greater than $+110$ degrees in adults

Right axis deviation of greater than $+120$ degrees in the young

S_1, S_2, S_3 pattern in children

Late intrinsicoid deflection in V_1 and V_2

Incomplete RBBB pattern in V_1 (rSr')

ST segment depression with upward convexity and inverted T waves in V_1 and V_2 and in the limb leads, with tall R waves

Reversal of precordial lead R wave progression

"Strain" pattern in V_1, V_2, II, III, and aV_F

Tall, peaked P waves in leads II, III, and aV_F and sometimes in V_1 (right-atrial involvement)

Associated right-atrial enlargement

Murphy has formulated two methods for identifying right-ventricular hypertrophy*:

Method 1 (59% sensitivity, 86% specificity); positive if one of the following is present:

1. R/S ratio in V_5 or V_6 is 1
2. S in V_5 or V;6 is 7 mm
3. Right axis deviation of $+90°$
4. P-pulmonale

Method 2 (40% sensitivity, 97% specificity); positive if any two of the above are present

Causes

▪ Mitral stenosis
▪ Chronic lung disease
▪ Atrial setpal defect
▪ Tetralogy of Fallot
▪ Pulmonary stenosis
▪ Tricuspid insufficiency

*From Murphy, M.E., et al: Reevaluation of electrocardiographic criteria for left, right, and combined cardiac ventricular hypertrophy, Am. J. Cardiol. **53:**1140, 1984.

Nursing Implications

The causes of right-ventricular overload are not as common as the causes of left-ventricular overload, and the fully developed ECG pattern is not often seen.

The nursing care is determined by the cause.

Variations

None

Differential Diagnosis

See ''Causes.''

Treatment

That of the primary disease

Left-Atrial Enlargement
Pathophysiology and Mechanism

Same as for left-ventricular hypertrophy

ECG Characteristics

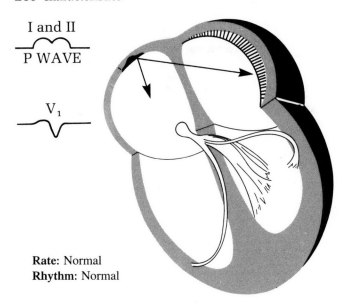

I and II

P WAVE

V_1

Rate: Normal
Rhythm: Normal

PR interval: Normal
QRS complex: Often that of left-ventricular hypertrophy
Distinguishing features: P wave (P-mitrale):
1. Widened to 0.12 sec or more
2. Notched with 0.04 sec between peaks
3. Deep broad negative terminal trough in V_1
4. May be negative in III and aV_F

Causes

▪ Those of left-ventricular hypertrophy

Variations

None

Differential Diagnosis

None

Treatment

That of the primary disease

Right-Atrial Enlargement
Pathophysiology and Mechanism

Same as for right-ventricular hypertrophy

ECG Characteristics

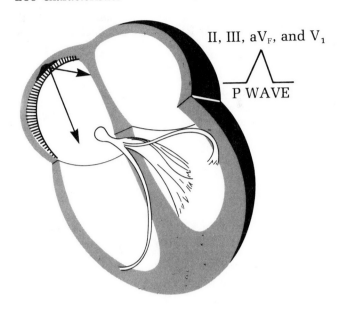

II, III, aV$_F$, and V$_1$

P WAVE

Rate: Normal

Rhythm: Normal

PR interval: Normal

QRS complex: qR in V$_1$ in the absence of myocardial infarction; diminished voltage in V$_1$ with threefold or more increase in V$_2$

Distinguishing features:

Tall peaked P waves in II, III, and aV$_F$ and sometimes in V$_1$ (P-pulmonale)

P wave axis to the right of $+70$ degrees (in chronic lung disease)

Causes

■ Those of right-ventricular hypertrophy

Variations

None

Differential Diagnosis

Left-atrial enlargement. If the right atrium enlarges enough to extend toward the left, the P waves of right-atrial enlargement may be inverted in V_1, simulating left-atrial enlargement.

Treatment

That of the primary disease

Potassium, Calcium, and the ECG

12

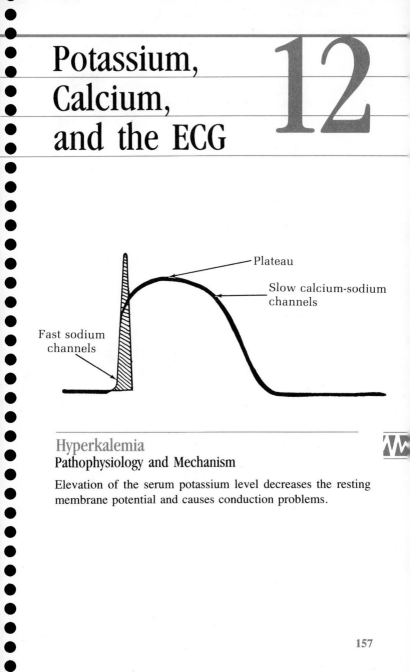

Plateau

Slow calcium-sodium channels

Fast sodium channels

Hyperkalemia
Pathophysiology and Mechanism

Elevation of the serum potassium level decreases the resting membrane potential and causes conduction problems.

ECG Characteristics

K⁺ 6.8

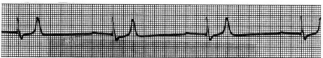

K⁺ 7.3

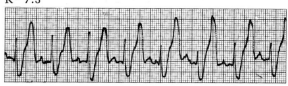

Sine wave: a terminal event

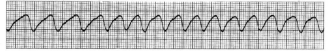

Rate: Normal

Rhythm: Normal

PR interval: Normal but P wave disappears as level of potassium rises

QRS complex: Widens

Distinguishing features: Early signs are tall peaked T waves, loss of ST segment, left axis deviation, wide QRS

P wave of low amplitude or barely visible

Serum K⁺ (mEq/L)

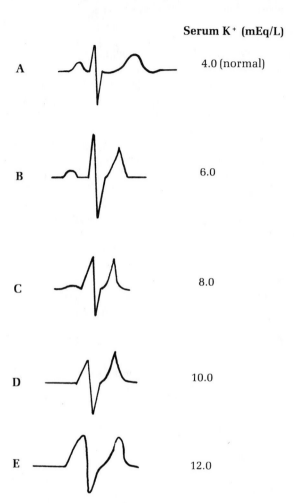

A   4.0 (normal)

B   6.0

C   8.0

D   10.0

E   12.0

5.5 mEq/L: T wave peaks
6.5 mEq/L: QRS widens; P wave is wide and of low amplitude
10   mEq/L: QRS slurred and wider; P wave barely visible
12   mEq/L: P wave has disappeared

Cause

- Kidney failure (most common cause)

Nursing Implications

This condition is potentially lethal but readily reversible; therefore, early diagnosis is imperative.

There is no constant association between an absolute potassium level and the ECG; the rate of progression of cardiac toxicity is variable, and signs and symptoms not uniformily present. Therefore, maintain a high index of clinical suspicion, especially in patients with anoxia, acidosis, trauma to soft tissues, oliguria, or a history of spironolactone or triamterene ingestion.

Treatment

The choice of treatment depends on the severity of the hyperkalemia. The patient is constantly monitored on the ECG.

Hypertonic Na^+ and Ca^{++} are indicated only if toxicity is advanced at time of discovery. They suppress the effects of hyperkalemia without affecting the potassium concentration.

Sodium bicarbonate in the presence of systemic acidosis lowers the serum potassium level by promoting cellular uptake.

Glucose and insulin promote uptake of potassium into liver and muscle cells.

Sorbitol and polystyrene sulfonate resin lower the total body potassium by cationic exchange.

Dialysis

Hypokalemia
Pathophysiology and Mechanism

At first hypokalemia causes an increase in the resting membrane potential (it becomes more negative), but this is soon followed by an increase in phase 4 depolarization in Purkinje fibers, which produces spontaneous ectopic beats and a resting maximal diastolic potential that becomes less and less negative until the fibers are nonexcitable. As the giant U wave appears the patient is vulnerable to torsades de pointes.

ECG Characteristics

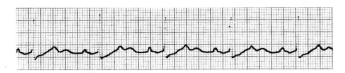

Rate: Normal
Rhythm: Normal
PR interval: Lengthens
QRS complex: Widens
Distinguishing features: The U wave gets taller and taller and fuses with the T wave.

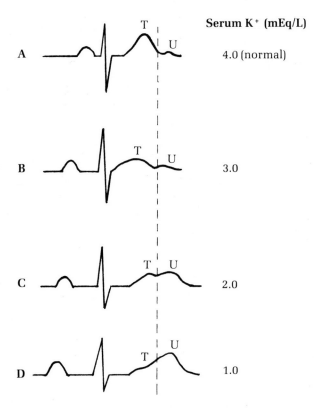

4 mEq/L: Normal U wave is same polarity as the T and of low amplitude

3 mEq/L: T and U same amplitude

2 mEq/L: U taller than T

1 mEq/L: Giant U wave fuses with the T

Causes

- Diuretics
- Vomiting
- Gastric suction

Nursing Implications

The diagnosis is made because of the ECG picture, the symptoms of polyuria in mild cases, and muscle weakness in more severe cases.

In the digitalized patient, even slight hypokalemia may precipitate serious arrhythmias.

Treatment

The route of repletion depends on the severity of the hypokalemia. The oral route is used in mild to moderate uncomplicated hypokalemia.

Hypercalcemia
Pathophysiology and Mechanism

ECG changes resulting from changes in serum calcium levels are of clinical importance only when they are extremely high or low. Calcium exerts itself on the plateau of the action potential (phase 2). Thus the length of the QT interval is inversely related to serum calcium concentration: hypercalcemia shortens the QT interval.

ECG Characteristics

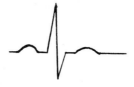

QT shortens

Rate: Normal
Rhythm: Normal
PR interval: Normal
QRS complex: Normal
Distinguishing features: Short QT interval (not always a reliable sign)

Causes

- Malignancy
- Vitamin D intoxication
- Sarcoidosis
- Primary hyperparathyroidism
- Milk-alkali syndrome
- Thyrotoxicosis
- Adrenal insufficiency
- Vitamin A intoxication
- Idiopathic hypercalcemia in infants
- Immobilization
- Immobilization
- Renal failure

Nursing Implications

Severe hypercalcemia is life threatening.
If the patient is taking digitalis, intoxication may result.

Treatment

The cause is treated and calcium excretion promoted.

Hypocalcemia
Pathophysiology and Mechanism

Since the length of the QT interval is inversely related to serum calcium concentration, hypocalcemia lengthens it. This lengthening of the refractory period as reflected in the QT interval is homogeneous, so that hypocalcemia rarely causes arrhythmias unless it is complicated by hypokalemia.

ECG Characteristics

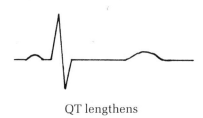

QT lengthens

Rate: Normal
Rhythm: Normal
Pr interval: Normal
QRS complex: Normal
Distinguishing features: Long QT interval

Causes

- Hypoparathyroidism
- Hypomalacia in adults and rickets in children
- Chronic steatorrhea
- Pregnancy
- Diuretics, such as furosemide or ethacrynic acid
- Respiratory alkalosis and hyperventilation
- Hypomagnesemia, possibly secondary to release of parathyroid hormone

Nursing Implications

The cause of the deficiency must be identified and treated. A thorough history and physical is indicated.

Treatment

The cause is treated and calcium replaced.

The Electrically Sensitive Patient

13

The primary reason for the increased shock hazard in critical care areas is the use of transvenous intracardiac catheters, which provide a direct electrical connection to the myocardium. Such a direct connection of the heart to the outside environment creates an electrically sensitive patient. Because the cardiac tissue is directly exposed, the patient is rendered extremely vulnerable to a level of electrical shock that is imperceptible to a person without a cardiac catheter.

Various studies have been made on the effect of electrical shock on both humans and dogs, and the results of some of these studies are summarized in Table 13-1.

Typical Conductors
Ionic Conductors

1. Saline
2. Urine
3. Blood
4. Coffee, soda, and so on

Metallic Conductors

1. Pacing catheters
2. Catheter metal guide wires
3. Thermodilution catheters
4. Metal furniture, bed lights, and instruments

Table 13-1 Effect of shock current on the heart

Current	Through Intact Skin (Macroshock)	Direct Contact to Myocardium (Microshock)
10 A	⎫ Sustained myocardial contraction	
5 A	⎬	
2 A	⎪	
1 A	⎭	
500 mA	⎫ Ventricular fibrillation (respiration continues)	
200 mA	⎬	
100 mA	⎭	
50 mA	Pain, fainting, exhaustion	
20 mA	Let go current (muscle contraction)	
10 mA		
5 mA	Maximum harmless current	
2 mA		
1 mA	Threshold of perception	Ventricular fibrillation (humans) (2.5 cm. diam. plate electrode)
500 µA		
200 µA		Ventricular fibrillation (humans) (0.25 cm. diam. plate electrode)
100 µA		Ventricular fibrillation in dogs (catheter)
50 µA		
20 µA		
10 µA		Maximum current recommended for electrically safe areas*
5 µA		

*Association for Advancement of Medical Instrumentation (AAMI), type A.

Sources of Currents

The basic source of all hazardous currents in the CCU is the electrical power available at the wall receptacle.

Leakage current is the most probable source of current dangerous to the electrically sensitive patient. Leakage current will seek any path from its metal case or parts to ground and increases in a humid environment and when subjected to moisture, dust, or a corrosive atmosphere. Leakage current is conducted harmlessly to the ground if the metallic case of the piece of equipment is connected by a separate wire in the line cord to the ground pin of the outlet.

Faults are actual malfunctions of equipment, whereby an internal conductor comes in contact with another conductor or with the case.

Hazardous Situations

Ungrounded Equipment

An epicardial or endocardial electrode or a cardiac pressure monitoring catheter, through the associated monitor, provides

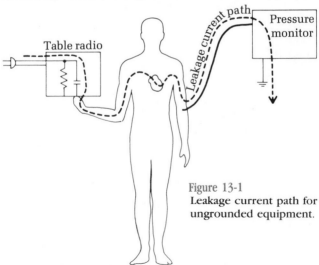

Figure 13-1
Leakage current path for ungrounded equipment.

a resistance to ground that is sufficiently low to allow a leakage current of an ungrounded table radio to pass through the heart if contact is made with the conductive case of the radio (Fig. 13-1).

Equipment with Defective Ground

A defective ground on an electric bed, for example, would allow a dangerous current to flow through the patient's heart if an attendant were to touch the bare pacemaker terminal while holding the bed rail (Fig. 13-2).

Nursing Implications

The nurse must avoid becoming part of a circuit that could allow current to flow through him or her and then through the

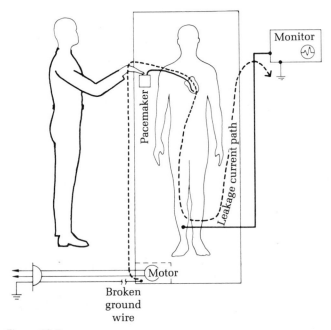

Figure 13-2
Attendant as part of leakage current path.

patient. The following measures will help to avoid such a potentially fatal situation:

1. Be aware that pressure catheters and endocardial or epicardial electrode wires in place provide a direct electrical connection to the patient's heart.
2. Insulate all metal terminals, guide wires, and uninsulated electrode wires as follows:
   a. Place plastic or rubber sleeving over exposed terminals.
   b. Wear surgical gloves whenever it is necessary to handle bare electrode wires or terminals.
   c. Place external battery-powered pacemakers in a surgical glove or plastic sheet to insulate their terminals.
3. When taking an intracardiac electrocardiogram, be certain that the intracardiac wire is connected to the V lead and not to the indifferent (right-leg) electrode.
4. Be aware that intraesophageal and intratracheal devices, because of their proximity to the posterior myocardium, present a hazard almost as great as that of intracardiac catheters and should be treated with the same care.
5. Maintain a continuing survey of the condition of equipment within the unit.
   a. If a tingling sensation (mild electrical shock) is felt when a piece of equipment is touched, it is an indication that the equipment is defective and poses a definite shock hazard to the patient. If not required for life support, the equipment should be removed from the area and tagged to alert others to the danger. When it is required for life support, it should be repaired (or, preferably, replaced) as soon as possible.
   b. The conditions of all power cords and plugs should be noted. The hospital electrician should repair or replace all frayed or damaged cords. Any equipment using two-pronged plugs should be removed *from the hospital* until the plugs can be replaced with the three-pronged grounding type.
6. Do not allow patient-supplied appliances in the unit un-

less they are battery-powered and not connected to the AC power.

7. Do not run heavy wheeled equipment over power cords, thus damaging them.

8. Do not store equipment in a manner that exposes the power cords to kinking or extremes of temperature.

9. Avoid the use of extension cords if at all possible.

   a. Two-wire extension cords defeat the grounding scheme of the equipment.

   b. If the use of an extension cord is absolutely necessary, it must be the three-wire type and it must be inspected often for an intact ground wire. If possible, such an extension cord should be dedicated to a specific piece of equipment and inspected with that equipment.

10. The appearance of AC interference on an ECG tracing can result from several causes. Some of these pose a hazard to the patient; others do not. In either event, the interference makes the tracing difficult to interpret, and the situation should be corrected at once. In an electrically safe area the usual cause of AC interference is dried out electrode pads or a defective patient cable. If neither of these is the case, the cause may be poorly grounded or defective electrical equipment in use on the patient. Through systematic disconnecting and reconnecting of each piece of eqiupment until the interference disappears, the offending piece of equipment can be identified. Since the presence of AC interference can indicate a shock hazard, equipment causing such interference should be removed from the unit and repaired.

11. Ensure that the redundant green ground wires often found on electric beds, ECG monitors, and other equipment used around electrically sensitive patients are plugged into the wall ground jacks.

12. Know the electrical safety program of your hospital, and become familiar with the instrument inspection schedule. Do not use equipment that has not been inspected in a reasonable amount of time or that is not intended for use around electrically sensitive patients.

13. Do not hesitate to report equipment that is operating erratically, producing a strange odor, tripping line-isolation monitors or circuit breakers, or performing in an abnormal manner.

14. Make sure that all equipment being used with a single patient is plugged into adjacent receptacles.

Artificial Cardiac Pacing

14

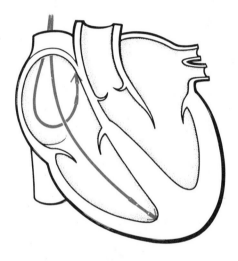

The Pacing System

The pacing system consists of a pulse generator and a lead electrode. The pulse generator contains the pacemaker electronics and the energy source for generating electrical stimuli; it is encased in a stainless steel or titanium housing that is hermetically sealed under a dry helium-and-air mixture to isolate the contents from the biological environment. The lead electrode, which may be unipolar or bipolar, is attached by a wire to the pulse generator.

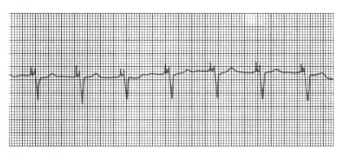

Figure 14-1
Bipolar pacemaker spike.

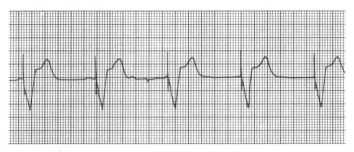

Figure 14-2
Unipolar pacemaker spike.

Bipolar systems have two electrodes in contact with cardiac tissue. The distal, or stimulating, electrode is usually the cathode. Fig. 14-1 shows the spike from a bipolar system.

A unipolar system has a negative electrode in contact with the heart and a positive extracardiac (indifferent) electrode, which is part of the pulse generator capsule. Fig. 14-2 shows the spike from the unipolar system. It is larger than that from the bipolar system and is thought to be more suitable for intracardiac sensing.

The Sensing Circuit

The sensing circuit detects intrinsic electrical impulses and inhibits generator discharge in their presence. Normally an electrical impulse of 2 mV or more is transmitted to the sensing circuit, and the pacemaker's output impulse is inhibited and the cycle reset.

Pacemaker Refractory Period

The refractory period of a ventricular pacemaker is the period during which a pulse generator is unresponsive to an input signal of specified amplitude. The refractory period ensures that the pacemaker does not sense its own R or T wave.

The refractory period of an atrial pacemaker is that time during which signals at the atrial input are ignored; this time begins when atrial or ventricular activity is sensed and ends at a programmed time in accordance with the patient's ventriculoatrial (VA) conduction so that retrograde P waves are ignored.

Hysteresis

Hysteresis, a feature of some pulse generators, provides a difference in time between the escape interval and the pacing interval. The escape interval is longer than the pacing interval, so that the pulse generator may not escape and pace the heart until the rate has dropped below about 60 pulses per minute (ppm). Once initiated, however, the pacing rate is about 72 ppm. This is illustrated in Fig. 14-3.

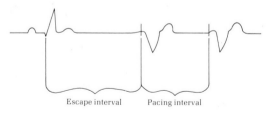

Escape interval   Pacing interval

Figure 14–3

Five-Position Pacemaker Code

The five-position pacemaker code of the Intersociety Committee on Heart Disease (ICHD) is universally used to describe pacemaker operation, with the first three positions being used most often. The first three positions are as follows. The fourth and fifth positions, not described here, indicate programmability and tachyarrhythmia functions.

1 Chamber Paced	2 Chamber Sensed	3 Mode of Response
V = Ventricle	V = Ventricle	I = Inhibited
A = Atrium	A = Atrium	T = Triggered
D = Dual (atrium and ventricle)	D = Dual (atrium and ventricle)	D = Dual (atrial triggered and ventricular inhibited)
O = None	O = None	R = Reverse
		O = None

The Pacing Modes
VVI Pacing

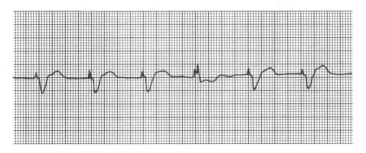

In the past, the most popular type of pacemaker was that with the VVI mode (ventricular-demand pacemaker). In the VVI mode, pacing and sensing occur only in the ventricle; this is the chamber that is evaluated when pacing function is assessed. Intrinsic ventricular activity will inhibit pulse generator output. Because sensing and pacing occur only in the ventricle, VVI pacing is appropriate only when there is no significant atrial contribution to cardiac output, as in atrial fibrillation. Such pacing is contraindicated in pacemaker syndrome or in congestive heart failure.

AAI Pacing

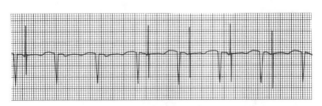

In the AAI mode, pacing and sensing occur only in the atrium, and the pacemaker is inhibited by sensed atrial activity. This type of pacemaker is appropriate only when AV conduction is adequate.

VDD Pacing

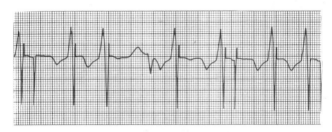

In VDD pacing, atrial activity is sensed and the ventricle is paced in synchrony. Pacing occurs only in the ventricle, but sensing occurs in both chambers. The pacemaker is triggered by intrinsic atrial activity and inhibited by intrinsic ventricular activity. If the intrinsic atrial rate falls below the programmed ventricular rate, only the ventricle will be paced. In such a case the pacemaker functions in the VVI mode. Such pacing is appropriate when AV conduction is not intact and ventricular pacing is necessary.

DVI Pacing

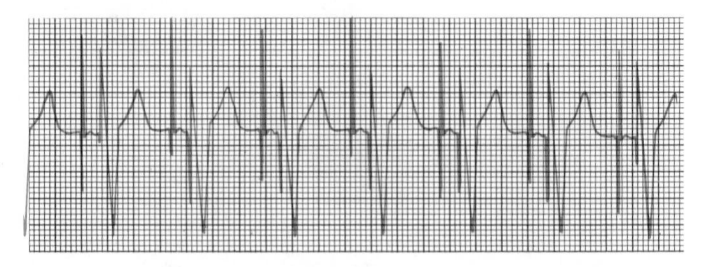

The DVI mode is dual-chamber pacing. Pacing occurs in either the atrium or the ventricle, or in both, but sensing occurs only in the ventricle. The pacemaker is inhibited by intrinsic ventricular activity.

DDD Pacing

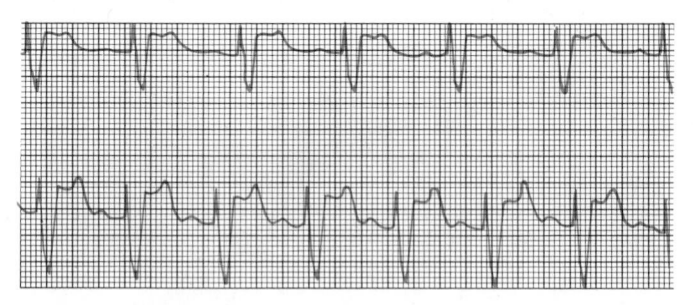

The DDD mode provides another form of dual-chamber pacing; pacing and sensing occur in either the atrium or the ventricle, or in both. Atrial or ventricular output is inhibited by sensed atrial or ventricular activity, and ventricular output is triggered by sensed atrial activity.

The DDD pacemaker has the potential to operate in four modes (VVI, AAI, VDD, and DVI), adapting to the patient's rhythm. Such a pacemaker would be totally inhibited by the patient's normal sinus rhythm. However, if there were sinus bradycardia, it would pace the atrium (AAI); if there were prolonged or blocked AV conduction, it would pace both the atrium and the ventricle sequentially (DDD).

The Pacemaker Syndrome

The pacemaker syndrome is weakness or syncope related to adverse hemodynamic effects of ventricular pacing. The causes are loss of atrial kick and simultaneous atrial and ventricular contraction.

Indications for Permanent Cardiac Pacemaker Implantation

Permanent cardiac pacemaker implantation in the treatment of bradyarrhythmias is justified, even if the patient is asymptomatic, when the AV block is at the level of the bundle branches and manifesting as type II second-degree or complete AV block.

In all other clinical settings the following conditions must be met before permanent pacing can be instituted:

1. Drugs must be excluded as a cause of conduction or impulse generation problems.
2. The patient must be experiencing serious symptoms as a result of failure of impulse generation or conduction.

For a detailed list of conditions requiring permanent pacing and conditions in which permanent pacing is not necessary, the reader is referred to the recent report of a highly qualified independent study group.*

Indications for Temporary Pacing

Indications for temporary pacing include the following:

1. Following open heart surgery
2. During cardiac catheterization or surgery
3. Before implantation of permanent pacemaker
4. Anterior-wall myocardial infarction with RBBB and left-anterior hemiblock or concurrent LBBB

*Phibbs, B., et al.: Indications for pacing in the treatment of bradyarrhythmias, JAMA 252(10):1307, 1984.

5. Acute inferior myocardial infarction with refractory complete AV block and ventricular ectopics and/or hemodynamic deterioration
6. Termination of atrial flutter, PSVT, or ventricular tachycardia
7. Electrophysiologic studies

Complications

Complications of pacing include electrode dislodgment, sensing or pacing failure, false sensing, failure to capture, endocardial puncture, and endless-loop tachycardia.

Electrode Dislodgment

Electrode dislodgment is the most frequent problem in temporary transvenous pacing and may result in sensing or pacing failure. If there is electrode dislodgment and a change in catheter position, the shape of the ventricular complex will change. Therefore, the expected ECG pattern should be noted and checked.

Sensing Failure

If electrode dislodgment and displacement are enough to break the generator's sensing circuit, the pacemaker will perform like a fixed-rate pacemaker, competing with the patient's intrinsic rhythm or competing with PVCs (Fig. 14-4).

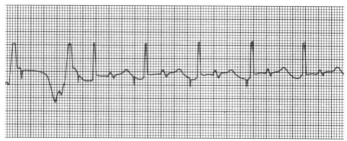

Figure 14-4
Sensing failure. The pacemaker fails to sense the patient's intrinsic rhythm and fires on the T waves of four complexes.

False Sensing

False sensing may be caused by drifting of the catheter toward the tricuspid valve with the resultant inhibition of discharge because of the sensing of atrial activity. In such a case, the pacemaker should be converted from the demand to the fixed-rate mode until the catheter can be repositioned. If the pacemaker is sensing ST segment elevations or T waves (as sometimes occurs with temporary pacemakers), the sensitivity of the external generator should be altered by turning the dial on the face of the unit toward the fixed-rate mode.

Failure to Capture

Failure to capture is illustrated in Fig. 14-5. Capture may be restored by increasing the milliampere output. If the magnitude of the pacemaker deflection is adequate for capture and it still does not take place, electrode displacement may be the cause.

Endocardial Puncture

Endocardial puncture results in cessation of pacing. If the patient is taking anticoagulants, cardiac tamponade may result. Endocardial puncture is confirmed by obtaining a unipolar electrogram from the distal electrode. This is done by connecting the V lead to the tip electrode (cathode). If the electrode is situated in the right-ventricular apex, the QRS com-

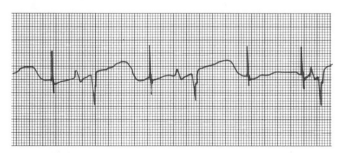

Figure 14-5

plex will be negative and the ST segment elevated (Fig. 14-6, *A*). If the endocardium has been perforated and the electrode is within the pericardial sac, the QRS will be positive, the ST segment depressed, and the T wave inverted (Fig. 14-6, *B*).

Endless-Loop Tachycardia

Endless-loop, pacemaker-mediated tachycardia is initiated when a retrograde P wave is sensed by a dual-chamber pacemaker, which in turn activates the ventricular pacemaker. If there is retrograde conduction from each ventricular beat and if the retrograde P wave reaches the atrium after the atrial refractory period and the pacemaker ventricular refractory period, an endless-loop tachycardia will ensue (Fig. 14-7). This

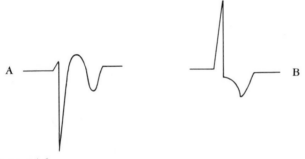

Figure 14-6
A, Pattern when the electrode is in the right-ventricular apex. **B,** Pattern when the electrode has perforated the myocardium and is in the pericardial sac.

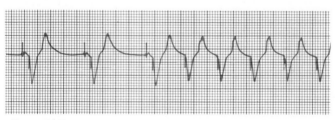

Figure 14-7

may be avoided by programming an adequate atrial refractory period. In this way the retrograde P wave is not sensed.

One way to terminate such a tachycardia is to switch to a DVI mode, thus eliminating atrial sensing.

Evaluating a DDD Tracing

Evaluate the Atrial Event

1. Is a P wave present?
2. Is it paced or intrinsic?
3. What is the rate of the atrial event?

Evaluate AV Delay

The AV delay is programmable and is the time between atrial and ventricular activity during which the pacemaker is "looking for" an R wave.

1. Is there a programmed AV delay?
2. What is its value?
3. Is it the same as in the tracing?

Evaluate the Ventricular Event

1. Are there intrinsic or paced ventricular complexes?
2. At what rate?
3. Has intrinsic ventricular activity been sensed?

Evaluate the VA Interval

The VA interval is determined by subtracting the AV delay from the programmed pulse interval. During part of this time, sensing for atrial activity takes place. This interval is functioning normally if intrinsic ventricular activity resets the VA interval.

Index

Page numbers followed by *t* indicate
tables.